# —YOUR—
# HEALTHCARE
# Playbook

## Winning the Game of Modern Medicine

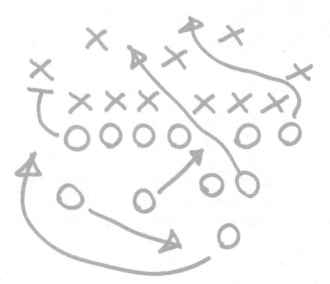

# Dennis Deruelle, MD, FHM

A SAVIO REPUBLIC BOOK

Your Healthcare Playbook:
Winning the Game of Modern Medicine
© 2017 by Dennis Deruelle, MD, FHM
All Rights Reserved

ISBN: 978-1-68261-242-2
ISBN (eBook): 978-1-68261-243-9

Cover Design by Quincy Avilio
Interior Design and Composition by Greg Johnson/Textbook Perfect

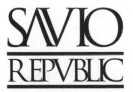

Published in the United States of America

# ACKNOWLEDGMENTS

This book would not have happened but for the sacrifice, patience, and hard work of some very important people. First and foremost, my wife Erin. She understands the essence of love and that is how my dreams come to life. I want to thank my wonderful children: Daniel, Nicholas, Joshua, Cecilia, Emily, and my step-daughter, Ryann. They all did their part not only by sacrificing time away from me, but also by listening through the many hours I spent regaling them with this topic! Nicholas, in particular, gave more than that—he was a sage counsel and used his burgeoning skills as a professional editor to help streamline and smooth parts of the book. I want to thank the members of my family, particularly my mother, father, sisters, aunts, and uncles, and friends for being good sports in letting me share some of their personal stories in the name of teaching. I also want to recognize those of my family who are no longer with us, some due to medical errors—if we can learn from their experiences, their loss will not have been in vain. Finally, without the wisdom, guidance, and encouragement, not to mention unparalleled editing skills of writer Garth Sundem, this book would have died many times. I enjoyed every minute of our collaboration.

A special thanks to Joel Osteen for introducing me to the firm of Dupree Miller and to what became my publisher, Post Hill Press. Thank you for believing in me.

# TABLE OF CONTENTS

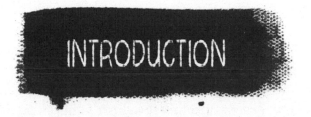

# INTRODUCTION

I became a doctor to help people. I wrote this book to empower them. After medical school, I thought treating diseases mattered most. After 20 years in practice I realize patients need much more. Their diseases, at times, are not their greatest foes. Many patients need a way through the confusing mess of paperwork, decisions, and insurance before and after we help them and send them on their way.

As you will read in these pages, my passion for helping patients navigate our confusing, inefficient, expensive, and sometimes dangerous health system is more than just professional—it's personal. My cousin Katie left the hospital after cancer surgery and died two weeks later without adequate clot-preventing medication. My mother's mismanaged complications after toe surgery left her with a permanently disfigured foot. Similar mismanagement left my father with irreversible neurologic damage. My sister's glee at the promise of affordable insurance through the Affordable Care Act was matched only by her disappointment after choosing a bad plan. Then there was a dying friend's doctor who indignantly asked me why she would want a second opinion. It's a long history—my grandmother struggled to afford my father's diabetes medicine and, after a missed diagnosis, my son performed CPR in vain on his dying stepfather. And this is a doctor's family! You might think that having an expert on call 24/7 would make my family immune to medical errors, misdiagnosis, insurance SNAFUs, and surgery complications. Nope. Far from it. Now after 20 years of practice, I have seen that no one is immune to the challenges and dangers of our medical system.

For every tragedy, however, there has been a victory that offers hope. A bout of colitis saved my father's life. Another surgery cured my mother. A brilliant doctor instantly spotted my uncle's symptoms of aneurysm. I have helped point family and friends toward cures for leukemia and lung cancer and have helped steer patients and my family to insurance choices that made treatment not only possible, but affordable. I have helped patients with their bills and have worked to troubleshoot ways to afford medications. I have been so honored throughout my career to have the information that patients, family, and friends needed.

Throughout my 20-year career I have worked in every setting from the ER to urgent care to primary care to hospitals to skilled nursing facilities to nursing homes and rehabs. I have been on healthcare teams ranging from huge, multi-specialty groups to a solo practice. I have been Chief Resident at a major academic medical center and a National Medical Director for one of the largest doctors' groups in the nation. I have traveled the U.S. fixing broken hospitals and healthcare systems. Then came the Affordable Care Act. I read every page and have led my organization in understanding the new, value-based models of healthcare. Now I'm working with my family, my friends, my organization, and my community to predict, understand, and navigate whatever is next in healthcare during this time of great political and social change.

Recently I started to think, *What if I could do for everyone what I do for my patients, family, and organization?* What if I could help not just these people that I talk with all the time, but help *everyone* understand how to navigate healthcare in a way that makes sense for safety, quality, and cost? For a while it seemed impossible or at least improbable—who wants to read a 1,000-page book on healthcare policy and who is willing to put in the brainpower needed to understand the ins and outs of how the ACA has transformed the insurance industry and which parts are likely to last? Not anyone I know, that's for sure.

Then I started thinking about my other love, football. With its agents, coaches, stadiums, contracts, trainers, positions, teams, data, and technology, the NFL is one of the few entities that can hold a candle to the complexity of healthcare. The important part is that while healthcare is confusing, many of us have a pretty good handle on how the NFL works. Healthcare is boring, but the NFL reaches 160 million fans, dominates all TV ratings, and has turned a weekend in February into a national holiday. I realized the NFL could be the Rosetta Stone that could help people translate and eventually win the game of medicine.

I'm an expert in healthcare, but before starting this book, I couldn't claim to be an expert in football. Sure, I had played in high school and continued as a super fan as an adult. But in order to pick apart how the NFL could help us understand healthcare, I needed to know more than the forward-facing aspects of the game. So I did what anyone would do—I emailed Roger Goodell. The next thing I knew, I was shaking his hand at the annual owners' meeting. My research took me from NFL headquarters on Park Avenue in Manhattan, to Lambeau Field, to Atlanta Falcon headquarters, to media days at the Super Bowl, along the way talking with NFL players, executives, doctors, marketers, and many more.

My mashup of football and healthcare would have one final prescient twist. In 1983, a New York business tycoon surprised the USFL, a fledgling professional football league, by buying the New Jersey Generals. His name was Donald Trump. Now he is poised to determine the fate of not only our country but our three-*trillion*-dollar healthcare system. This book is meant use the NFL as a model to help you understand timeless issues in your use of healthcare. But trying to completely disentangle healthcare from politics would be like trying to play a football game without referees. The rules create the realities. For that reason, I added a short section exploring how a Trump administration may reshape the rules of healthcare, today, tomorrow, and in the many years to come.

What I have come to understand is that at the end of the day, no matter the rules and red tape and changing political realities, it is the stories behind the games of healthcare and the NFL that reach us and teach us. Behind these stories of patients and players, and of coaches and doctors, are simple and concise "plays" to help you cut through the red tape and find the most value in healthcare. I wrote this book because I had to. Honestly, it has been one of the hardest of my professional endeavors. Now I hope you'll use it to win the most important game of your life—the modern game of medicine. This is your playbook. Welcome to the team.

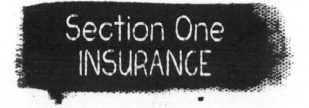

# Section One
# INSURANCE

Buying insurance is your first opportunity to make a game plan. Like an NFL team planning for next Sunday's game, you think about the challenges you're going to face and then decide how you will counter them. Then when you face these challenges, you know what to do—whether it's a young, healthy person who might break a leg or an older person planning for a chronic condition, choosing your health insurance is your opportunity to decide how, where, and from whom you will receive care.

The first time I made one of these plans was when I started med school. Like starting a new job, those few days before classes were filled with excitement and anxiety...and reams of paperwork. When you are signing promissory notes for loans that are larger than a home mortgage, health insurance costs are an afterthought. So I did what most American men do: I let my then-wife choose my plan for me. She was a nurse and so in addition to two plans offered by my school, we had a third choice from her employer. She signed us up for one of the school plans and that was that. As my second year began, signing to keep my same plan required even less thought. Done!

That year, my wife gave me the news that I was going to be a father. I was elated! And panicked! A father? I could barely manage my own life! Would I fail out of medical school?

But pregnancy is nine months long for a reason; it gives nervous dads time for the shock to wear off. Like all young expecting parents, we were soon caught up in preparations: the crib, the bouncer, the stroller, and so on. As it turned out, my wife would need a Cesarean section so instead of a surprise 2:00 AM sprint to the hospital, we chose a day and time for the delivery as if it were a hair appointment. Behind the scenes, our insurance company was busy authorizing everything we would need for the big day...or so we thought.

Checking into the hospital was just like checking into a hotel. We presented our cards and we were in. There are only so many moments when you gaze upon life's beauty in its purest form, and the birth of a child is one. Delirious from sleep deprivation and the joy of being a parent, we readied ourselves to check out. Then came the news: an employee from the business office visited our room to let us know that our hospital stay was not authorized. The company that carried our medical school insurance policy had dropped the plan. Just like that, we found ourselves without health insurance, looking at a $7,000 hospital bill.

"How would you like to handle the bill?" the business office representative asked politely. Oh, I handled it all right. Assuming it must be a mistake, I handled it right into the trashcan. It didn't take long for the collections letters to start.

All this is to say that my first attempt at making a healthcare game plan didn't go well. It was like knowing you're going to play the mid-2000s New England Patriots and prioritizing your run defense over rushing Tom Brady. You can do better. I realize picking your health plan ranks right up there with renewing your driver's license in the great pantheon of annoying things. However, it is one of those necessary evils that could literally save your life.

This section will explain the ins and outs of the different kinds of insurance plans, pointing out the things you will want to consider when choosing a plan. It will also explore how the rules that govern these plans are changing and may change to align with the goals of the Trump administration. But before reading about these plans and taking a quick and what I hope is relatively painless digression into politics, it's important to understand the language—at first, health insurance terms can be like a rookie trying to learn the playbook for the first time. Knowing the following terms is an essential step in determining which insurance plan is best for you:

## Insurance Terms

### PREMIUM

Your health insurance "premium" is the fixed amount of money you pay to the insurance company every month, quarter, or year. In exchange for your premium, your insurer agrees to accept some of the financial risk associated with your healthcare costs. If you have insurance through your employer, the premium is usually deducted directly from your paycheck and most employers help offset this cost (as one of its employee benefits). Both you and your employer pay insurance premiums with pre-tax dollars, making health insurance premiums a little cheaper.

## COST SHARING

When you use healthcare, you will pay part of the bill and your insurer will pay another part. Think of it like splitting the check at a restaurant. There are a couple ways that insurers determine the split, including some of the terms below.

## DEDUCTIBLE

I call this the *destructible* because unless you're careful, it can destroy your budget. This is the amount of money you must pay before your insurance kicks in. It's also one of the most confusing and frustrating terms in healthcare, and one of the biggest sources of OOPs! (out-of-

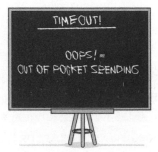

pocket spending). Depending on the plan, you may have different deductibles for family members, medications, and hospitalizations. A high-deductible plan comes with an attractive premium, but be aware that in this form of cost sharing, you may have to pick up the tab before your insurer starts helping with the bill.

## CO-PAY

This is the fixed amount you pay for certain aspects of your care, like medications or seeing your doctors. A co-pay is usually $5 to $40 dollars and is due at the time of your care. Doctors are not allowed to forgive a patient's co-pay, especially for Medicare. Your co-pay is always required and does not count towards your deductible.

## CO-INSURANCE

This is a percentage of your healthcare costs that you will pay after you have met your deductible and before you reach your out-of-pocket maximum.

## OUT-OF-POCKET MAXIMUM

This is the total amount you can be required to pay in one calendar year. Once you reach your out-of-pocket maximum, your insurer will pay 100 percent of your healthcare costs. As of 2017, the Centers for Medicare and Medicaid Services (CMS) sets the out-of-pocket maximum for individuals at $7,150 and for families at $14,300. These maximums will vary slightly for High Deductible and Health Savings Account plans.

## ESSENTIAL BENEFITS

All health insurance plans must cover the following ten *essential benefits*. Beyond these ten essential benefits, insurance plans may or may not cover things like cosmetic surgery and in-vitro fertilization.

- ▶ ambulatory patient services (non-hospital)
- ▶ emergency services
- ▶ hospitalizations
- ▶ maternity and newborn care
- ▶ mental health and substance abuse disorders services including behavioral health
- ▶ prescription drugs
- ▶ rehabilitative and habilitative services and devices
- ▶ laboratory services
- ▶ preventative services and chronic disease management
- ▶ pediatric services including oral and vision care

## FLEXIBLE SPENDING ACCOUNTS

This is an employer's plan in which an employee can set aside pre-tax dollars from his or her paycheck to pay premiums or medical expenses not covered by the plan. The employer may make contributions. It is customary to have a fixed period in which the funds must be used or you will lose them. You can carry $500 forward or have a grace period to use them; ask your employer.

## HEALTH SAVINGS ACCOUNTS

Like it sounds, this is a savings account for medical expenses funded by employees' pre-tax dollars with allowable contributions from employers. These accounts can roll over and be portable with different employers. Under ACA rules, you must select a high deductible plan to have an HSA and not be enrolled in Medicare or be claimed as a dependent on a tax return. However, the rules governing HSAs are likely to continue shifting during and after the Trump administration. How these rules will change depends on the prevailing political climate. Overall, Republicans tend to highlight the personal choice and that comes with saving and spending your own money, whereas Democrats tend to insist that only people with disposable incomes are *able* to put money aside in an HSA. In this time of shifting politics and changing regulations, keep your eyes on HSAs.

## GATEKEEPER

The healthcare professionals responsible for approving all treatments, tests, medications, and referrals.

## PRIOR AUTHORIZATION

Some medical benefits require advanced notice and approval from the insurer.

## INSURANCE APPEAL

When a claim is denied, the insured person may file an appeal that triggers the insurance company to take a second look. This appeal can be internal, within the insurer's review system, or external, usually involving third party arbitration as per the rules of the policy.

# A Note on Healthcare, Politics, and the Pace of Change

For me, the greatest allure of the NFL is its second-to-second unpredictability and the chance of a surprise ending—on any given Sunday, the saying goes, every two-touchdown underdog has the chance to beat the odds and knock off the favorite. That's certainly what happened in the 2016 election! Just as the results of games and elections may be unpredictable, so too is unpredictability a tool used in these contests. If a team runs the ball for every offensive play, the defense will wise up and learn to stop it. Unpredictability makes it hard for opponents to guess which plays will be called, which players will play, and how these plays and players fit into a team's overall game plan. Although President Trump makes use of this same unpredictability, we can see some patterns in his play-calling that help us guess at his game plan. Consider this short section like a scouting report: I have researched and studied his team and their plans, to make an informed guess about how the Trump team will affect healthcare, in the short-term and long after administrations inevitably change again. The good news is that the vast majority of the material in this book will be relevant regardless of which party holds the White House. Depending on your political views, you may consider it good news or bad news that many of the ideas put in place by the Affordable Care Act will almost certainly be slow to change as well. Here's why:

- ▶ As I outline in this section on health insurance, most of you are "drafted" into your employer's healthcare team. This was the case before the ACA and will remain the case during and after the Trump presidency. Changes to how these employer-sponsored plans are taxed have been proposed, but I doubt this will become a reality in the near future, and the anchor of health insurance linked with employment is unlikely to shift.

- ▶ The ACA will be repealed...but only certain parts of the systems it put in place will actually be unraveled. Replacement plans will phase in over years and will need bipartisan support.

- ▶ Large parts of the ACA designed to improve value in healthcare, like Patient-Centered Medical Homes (PCMHs), Accountable Care Organizations (ACOs), and Bundled Payments (BPCI) have been cemented in more recent bipartisan legislation.

There's another reason that many of the ACA systems will remain during and after Trump and that is the fact that some (but certainly not all!) of these systems are popular on both sides of the aisle. The following ACA provisions are likely to stick around because we like them:

- ▶ People with pre-existing conditions will continue to have some mandated access to health insurance, but this protection will likely be accomplished in a different manner than in the ACA.

▶ You will likely be able to keep your children on your insurance until they are age 26.

▶ For those who cannot afford insurance and even those that can, there will likely be some form of tax credit to offset some of your healthcare and insurance costs.

When I was a kid, we would argue for hours about whose NFL team was better. At some point, someone would invoke the fact that my team lost to theirs, to which I would astutely respond, "No, that day was opposite day, so my team actually won!" The ACA had winners and losers. The healthcare changes advocated by President Trump will be like opposite day, turning many of these losers into winners and, unfortunately, vice versa, winners into losers. Here are a few important examples:

▶ If you considered yourself on the losing side of the individual mandate, you will now win. The individual mandate will likely go away.

▶ Under the ACA, there was a mandate that employers offer insurance. Employers that considered themselves losers will win more freedom to choose how they offer insurance to their employees. (Of course, the employees who won the right to insurance under this mandate may lose.)

▶ In states that expanded Medicaid, millions of newly eligible patients won health insurance for the first time. Under new rules, they may lose this insurance.

- In states that didn't expand Medicaid, people who remained ineligible for Medicaid will likely win some kind of subsidy under future plans.

- The young and healthy who were incentivized through penalties to pay higher premiums under the ACA will likely get lower rates.

- The older and sicker patients who got lower premiums under the ACA will likely lose that advantage.

- If you felt the required essential benefits under the ACA were too broad, you will likely win the option to select more individualized plans with the ability to include and exclude benefits.

Perhaps even more important than some of these specifics are the principles that underlie President Trump's approach to health insurance and healthcare. Here are some broad themes that will shape the future under his leadership:

- Competition will replace regulation and penalties as the driver of value. You will have more choices in the future, and your dollars will determine which choices endure.

- You will have more out-of-pocket expenses (OOPs) but those of us able to store money in incentivized Health Savings Accounts (HSAs) will be able to offset many of these costs.

- HSAs will become more important for everyone regardless of age, income, or type of insurance, even for those enrolled in Medicaid or Medicare.

▶ You will have the ability to make your own value choices, and making the best choices will require more "comparency"—the ability to compare transparent services, plans, and options.

▶ Each state will have to choose how to distribute block grants for Medicaid, giving less care to more people, or more care to fewer people. Like patients, states will have more choice but also be forced to pay more of the bill.

▶ Health and wealth will remain tightly linked. The healthy will amass savings in growing HSA accounts and the unhealthy will have less to offset their ever-increasing costs.

▶ Individual accountability will make rewards like "Fitcoin" (my term for incentivized wellness programs) a great opportunity to lower your healthcare costs. On the other side, there will be more penalties for those of us unable to meet wellness goals.

In light of these changes associated with the Trump presidency, your best game plan is to keep half an eye on changing rules, but to focus more on the big principles of healthcare decision-making. Look to maximize quality and lower your cost to get the best *value*. When you have the chance to be a free agent, wielding the leverage of choice, take it—but be aware that you may pay for this privilege. When you have less choice, make your choices count by focusing on the parts of the system that are closest to you, namely your healthcare team. If the ACA exchanges are right for you, keep signing up until they change or go away. If you have Medicaid, keep it until your state comes up with other options. If you have employer-sponsored insurance, keep it until incentives and opportunities make it reasonable to be a free agent. Watch Medicare: You may have more options in the future to use Medicare funds toward a private plan. Take a note from President Trump's book and make deals when you can, especially as there becomes more space to negotiate agreements with doctors and hospitals.

Overall, remember that your game plan is a living document. An NFL team's playbook evolves as personnel and rules change and your healthcare playbook will have to evolve as well. Learning to use healthcare is an ongoing process, not something you chisel in stone, but something that you will optimize across your lifespan. I'm changing, too. Just as I read almost everything written about the ACA with you in mind, you can bet that I will be doing the same with all the changes that follow. And remember, the specifics change, but the ideas remain the same. By understanding the underpinnings of our healthcare system, you will continue to have the tools you need to find value. Quality divided by cost equals value. No political wrangling is going to change that.

# CHAPTER I:

## The MVP, Coaches, Owners & Agents of Your Healthcare Team

In 1983 when I was a freshman at the University of Texas at Austin, it wasn't hard to tell who was on the football team—players walked around campus wearing orange shirts with "TEAM" printed in huge letters and underneath it a lowercase "me." Unfortunately, I had a better chance of bleeding burnt orange blood than getting my hands on one of those shirts, let alone making the football team. But the message stuck with me: The "TEAM" was literally above the "me."

When I recently spoke with Rich McKay, president of the Atlanta Falcons, and, in my opinion, one of the NFL's best and brightest executives, I asked him if there is a secret to the NFL's success and he echoed the sentiment of the UT football shirts. He called this secret "league-think," which to him is the philosophy of putting the best interests of the league first. "The success of the NFL is in the forefathers realizing that to be successful, all teams from 1-to-32 must be successful," McKay said. For example, he noted the system of revenue-sharing between teams like the Packers and the Jets in which these teams with vastly different TV markets getting an equal share of profits. He said "league-think" is a philosophy and although there have been some tough votes to keep this prioritization of the league-before-teams, it has served them well. You see, the NFL is really a "team of teams"—one organization composed of many smaller organizations—and has put that big team of the league above all else.

Healthcare, on the other hand, is "teams of teams"—many organizations without, necessarily, one overarching team—making this kind of collaboration and integration much more difficult. In fact, healthcare is so fragmented it is like the components of its teams are not even in the same sport, like the NFL trying to communicate and coordinate with the NHL and MLB. This is an idea we'll come back to throughout this book, but basically football and healthcare are both composed of many teams, all of which work together with varying degrees of success. In healthcare, these teams include your family, an insurance organization, the many teams in a hospital, your primary care provider's office team, and many more. It's not just that "a team" needs to work together, but that widely diverse, individual teams need to interface and coordinate toward the goal of your health... all without dropping the ball. The NFL has done his beautifully—we see the game on Sunday, but behind the scenes is the massive infrastructure of an organization that puts its singular vision above any of its parts. The goal, simply, is to win, and the pursuit of this goal means that all the teams composed of many "me's" have to work together for the common good. For the NFL, this is relatively easy: all of its teams are under one business. And, in fact, healthcare may be moving toward this one-business model as well.

Still, the NFL isn't without alignment problems. Sometimes it's easy—think of a star quarterback who wants to set the single-season passing record. His coach recognizes the quarterback's talent and decides to highlight the passing game. The owner wants to sign a free agent wide receiver who can catch these throws. The stadium replaces grass with artificial turf, which will make the new receiver even faster. In this case, individual goals align with team goals, which all align with league goals. When this happens within a team, sports analysts call it *chemistry*.

Sometimes it's a little more difficult for the "me's" in the NFL to line up behind a team's best interests. You can probably think of an example. Take quarterback Kelly Stouffer who, after being picked in the first round of the 1987 draft by the St. Louis Cardinals, sat out the entire year with a contract dispute. The team went 7-8, missed the playoffs, and traded Stouffer to the Seattle Seahawks, where this promising pick had a short, undistinguished career. In football, when "me" comes before "TEAM," both suffer.

Healthcare is just beginning to understand how to work in teams. And like the NFL, sometimes all the "me's" have no problem working toward the same goals. Imagine you're admitted to the hospital for pneumonia. You want to get better fast and go home. Your doctor wants the same thing because she prides herself on practicing the best medicine possible. The hospital only gets paid a lump sum for your stay and so they want you to get better fast and go home as well. Your insurer has to pay the bill so they also want a short stay with no complications. See the chemistry?

The future of healthcare is being designed to find these sweet spots where all the "me's" win and thus so does the team. The problem is when the best interests of all these players on a healthcare team come into conflict. For example, recently my best friend called. His mother-in-law, Janet, had just been diagnosed with late-stage liver cancer. We all knew what this meant. My friend was calling because one doctor wanted Janet to do one thing and another doctor wanted her to do something else. Meanwhile, her insurance company kept delaying approval for tests and additional opinions, resulting in a mountain of paperwork and endless hours on hold. Three weeks had gone by since her diagnosis and there had been almost no movement. My friend asked if I would call his mother-in-law's doctor. When I did, the doctor said, "I don't understand why Janet is trying to get all these opinions—I already told her what to do!" If the doctor was this rude to me, I can't imagine what she was like with her patients! And it turned out that the doctor's staff had misunderstood the doctor's directions and had failed to send Janet's information to the National Cancer Institute for a remote second opinion. Insurer, office, doctor, patient: everyone was looking out for their own best interest (or bottom line) and no one was on the same team. By putting their own interests first, not only was the team dysfunctional, but for the "me," time was literally running out.

When an insurer puts money above your health, the results can be devastating. When doctors place their desire to get home sooner above their desire to offer a thorough examination, bad things happen. If a hospital chooses profit over effective medicine, your health suffers. In other words, this is one way that effective healthcare is opposite the NFL: In healthcare, "me" has to come before "team."

Now, I am around some of the best hospitals, doctors, and insurers in the country and I rarely see the needs of the team overtly trump those of a patient. No doctor drives into work motivated to put themselves above their patients. Hospitals spend thousands of hours in meetings trying to ensure excellent care. Insurers certainly need profits but in my meetings with them they are focused on doing the right thing by their patients. Is it always the case? No. And even in the best healthcare teams, small misalignments happen all the time.

This book is about learning how to make sure that "me" is above "Team" in your own healthcare and the care of people you love—and it is about recognizing when it's not and doing something about it! The first step is to understand how these systems work and what the roles of all the people who make up healthcare's many moving parts are. This chapter starts to break down the structure of this complex, multi-dimensional entity so that you can see inside the system to the places where you can get the most value. Throughout, we'll go back to the NFL to help you understand the new teams of healthcare and give you all the insider knowledge you need to make the most informed decisions for your health. First, let's meet your team!

## Patient = MVP and Star Quarterback

A few years ago, one of my sisters visited an orthopedic surgeon to discuss her back pain. The surgeon came into the room, gave a quick exam, asked a few questions, and within minutes he was outlining a plan as he headed out the door. In short, the surgeon was acting like the quarterback, calling the plays that my sister was supposed to run without question. But I had coached my sister the day before to tell the surgeon that she didn't just want to get by but that she wanted to return to running and to her athletic lifestyle. That day as the surgeon was leaving, she stopped him and said, "Aren't you interested in what I want? Don't you want to learn about me?"

He came back in the room and she explained that she wanted more than pain management. When he checked his watch several times she asked, "Is there somewhere you need to be?" Finally, he apologized and kept listening. When the surgeon finally understood, he changed the plan and ordered more X-rays. By acting like the team quarterback, my sister ensured that all her options would be on the table. Like her, you can call your own healthcare plays.

Vince Lombardi said, "Football is the perfect team game except for one glaring imbalance—the quarterback is too important." Healthcare isn't a perfect team, either: *You* are too important. You are the quarterback, the MVP, and healthcare's *raison d'etre*. When doctors and insurance companies and hospital executives talk about the "point of care," that's *you*.

Everything your healthcare team does should begin and end with you. It's your goals and preferences that should guide the plays for your team. NFL teams build around the quarterback as the foundation. Star quarterbacks determine the kind of offense, which players are drafted, the warm-up drills and even (sometimes…) the pressure of the footballs. Building the healthcare team around you as its quarterback is called, "Patient Centered Care." Unfortunately, this is a new system—too often, healthcare has been built around the hospitals, doctors, insurance companies, and other entities that would optimize the ease of care, cost of care, or speed

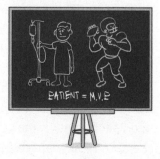

PATIENT = M.V.P

of care. This is changing and you need to be empowered to take your rightful position. *You need to claim your place as the quarterback of your healthcare team.* When the system isn't listening or you find yourself being shoved into the role of backup quarterback (or backup-backup special teams…), be like my sister and call a *timeout*! Make the "T" with your hands and start calling the plays. Be the quarterback. Be the MVP.

## Insurance Industry = NFL Owners

A woman I'll call Melissa had finally reached a time in her life when her children were raised and her career was flourishing. She traveled for her job, loving the freedom and constantly changing scenery. Then the pain started: severe, sharp pain radiating down her arms as if from one of Dante's lower circles of Hell. She tried physical therapy and exercise and injections all to no avail. After months of work, the pain continued. Confident in her orthopedic surgeon, together they decided it was finally time to alleviate the pressure on her neck nerves.

On her final office visit before surgery, the surgeon ordered a CT scan to take a final look at his target. He gave her a prescription slip for the scan, but when Melissa went to leave, the office clerk motioned for her to stop. "I'm so sorry," she said, cringing, "your insurer denied the CT scan. They said they would approve an MRI instead."

Bewildered, Melissa told her surgeon who said the MRI would be worthless. He insisted that Melissa would need a CT scan, which uses a series of X-rays to visualize bones (while an MRI is usually better for visualizing problems with soft tissues). "You will have to pay out of pocket," the clerk said.

With two days until surgery, everything was now on hold. We'll get back to Melissa later, but for now it's enough to see that insurance companies are a powerful member of your healthcare team. Chances are you already know this—*everyone* has a story of a procedure or a test denied, or contested claims, or an unexpected bill, or endless hoops to jump through before an insurer will cover a treatment that you and your doctor knew was best all along.

Like how the decisions of an NFL owner can dictate the fate of their team, an insurance company's decisions can control a large part of your healthcare destiny. Ideally, health insurers would be like NFL owners, deciding which tools to buy for their team, but always with the team's best interests in mind. That's not always the case.

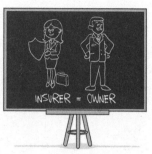

## Doctors = Coaches

The best coaches transcend their sideline role to play a much greater part in their players' lives. Witness Rice University running back Luke Turner, crying at a press conference while describing his coach, David Bailiff. Many players attribute their success on and off the field to their coaches. Doctors go into their profession hoping to have this kind of impact on patients' lives—to have the privilege of sharing the doctor–patient relationship, that sacred space where decisions of life and death and innermost secrets and fears are shared.

Luckily, as in football, your success can be your coach's success too. In the early days of the NFL, players and coaches were paid a standard fee per game—the more they played, the more they earned. It's a little different now; have you seen how much more coaches can make when they win? The way doctors are paid is changing too. Instead of earning a pure per-visit fee, now based on the Affordable Care Act and other forces, doctors are increasingly being paid based on the quality of their work. I call it "outcomes = incomes" and it's a paradigm-shifting transformation. It means that how you do will determine their pay.

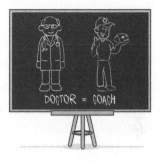

Coaches cannot play your game of health—that is, your life outside the office or hospital. They use their expertise to help call the plays but in the end the execution of these plays is largely up to you.

## Hospitals and Clinics = Stadiums and Facilities

If stadiums are where football happens, then hospitals and doctors' offices are the same for healthcare. This is where healthcare happens. And like a football stadium, the quality of the facility influences the overall quality of the care and the experience. Like stadiums, hospitals also have complex business relationships with their communities. Did you know that until 2015, the NFL was a 501(3)c nonprofit like many hospitals? Look around an NFL stadium—for whom does the announcer work? Who do the beer and peanut vendors report to? What about all those people in the press box? Like a sports stadium, hospitals have many teams with

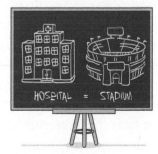

many coaches and many owners, some working for the hospital and others playing their part in your care while employed by themselves or by someone else. We assume that everyone in a stadium and everyone in a hospital works for the hospital or stadium "team." That's not the case and these settings are definitely a place to be aware of potential difficulties and conflicts that arise due to the challenges of working with "teams of teams."

## Parent, Spouse, Loved One, Caregiver, or Advocate = Agent

A while ago, I was in Dallas chatting with my wife on the phone as I waited for my flight home to Florida. She didn't mention anything unusual and we hung up planning to see each other in a couple hours. Then moments later, my stepdaughter, Ryann, called me back, concerned. My wife has had intermittent abdominal pain literally since the first day we met, but to Ryann this time it seemed...*different*. I spoke with my wife again and I agreed with Ryann: something was wrong. I instructed Ryann to take her to the ER and boarded the plane for one of the longest flights of my life.

Over the plane's WiFi, I learned that a section of my wife's colon had twisted. Ryann was giving me the play by play via email as I fired off what to say and do. The colon was dying and needed to come out. But at midnight when I arrived at the hospital, I learned the ER doctor was not convinced of the diagnosis. I pushed her: "Let's get the radiologist to make the call, and let's get a surgeon now to review the findings," I said. The surgeon came in about 4:00 AM and confirmed the diagnosis. My wife went into surgery within the hour. Later, looking at the CT scan together, this was not an on-the-fence kind of call. I was glad I pressed.

Then it turned out that the day after the successful surgery, her surgeon was leaving for Europe and had to turn my wife's care over to a colleague. At our first check-in, the replacement surgeon strode in and amid a room full of visitors casually sat down next to my wife, listened 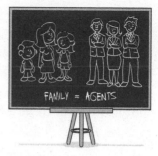 to her lungs briefly, and said that everything sounded good but that a chest X-ray showed a little nodule that would require follow-up with a CT scan. "Take care," he said and was out the door. I could see the horror on my wife's face: *Hey I can deal with losing part of my colon but lung cancer... what?*

I immediately chased the surgeon out in the hall and when he pulled up the report on the computer, I was able to see the nodule was far less ominous than he had made it sound— likely a small area of slightly less aerated lung that would go away after surgery. I was sure the CT scan would confirm that everything was fine. A day went by and then another...and finally I asked the replacement surgeon when he was planning to schedule the CT scan. "Oh," he said, "I forgot."

Needless to say, I was not amused. I was happy I had left my wife's side for only about an hour during her nine-day stay. Remember the 1990's movie *Jerry Maguire* when Cuba Gooding Junior's NFL character makes Tom Cruise's sports agent character yell, "Show me the money!" The athlete wanted to be sure the agent had his best interest firmly in mind. As the agent, Tom Cruise's job wasn't to care about coaches or owners or scouts—it was to have his players' backs. That's your job as the loved one of someone who needs healthcare. You're their agent. You're they're advocate. You've got their back.

And when you're in a healthcare setting there is nothing wrong with having your agent with you. Agents can be your family, friends or caregivers. Sadly, many patients have none of these advocates. Remember that CT scan the replacement surgeon forgot to order and that I assumed would show a fairly safe pattern of low lung aeration? Well, it came back positive for many blood clots in the lung, a complication of surgery that could have killed my wife. Without this test, she might have died. And without an advocate—her agent!—at her side in the hospital, this test could easily have slipped everyone's mind.

Now, these comparisons between roles in the NFL and roles on your healthcare team aren't perfect and they're not meant to be. They're meant to be inroads to understanding what these people and entities do—and how your role and motivations work with or, sometimes against, all the other members of your healthcare team. Now that you have a quick introduction to these roles—you're the MVP, insurers are owners, doctors are coaches, hospitals are stadiums, and loved ones are agents—you can use this understanding to influence how you use these people on your team. Work with your coach to call the plays. Let your agent be your advocate. Take into account the quality of the stadium when choosing which team to play for. And watch for ways this entire system does or doesn't put you, the MVP, first. Of course, we'll talk a lot more about all these things later—how to optimize these roles is central to getting the most from health insurance and healthcare. For now, think about the people and places that fill these roles on your own team. How are they like or unlike their NFL counterparts? Do you wish they would be more or less similar?

Again: The purpose of this book is to use something you know (the NFL) to help you understand something that's difficult to know (healthcare). Your understanding starts now.

# CHAPTER 2:
## Choosing Your Healthcare Team

"They told me my mammogram is abnormal. Please call me. Love you. Mom."

Do you remember old-fashioned answering machine messages? This is one I wish I could forget. At the time, I was an internal medicine resident at the University of North Carolina at Chapel Hill. I basically lived at the hospital. The few hours I was able to sneak away, my four young children (I would eventually have five and a step-daughter!) kept me plenty busy. Having raised four children herself, my mother was now busy realizing her dreams, living in sunny Florida and finishing college and then a master's degree.

By the time I checked the phone, the message was already a couple days old, but it hit me with an immediacy that made everything else fade away. "Abnormal" and "mammogram" may be the two scariest words a woman can hear and it's not that much better for her son who is a doctor. Every day, I saw the ravages of breast cancer in my hospital, one of the preeminent breast cancer research centers in the world.

I called her back immediately and she said, "I am fine! I found a nice surgeon. They have to biopsy this spot. How are the kids?"

"Wait, what do you mean you found a surgeon, Mom?" I knew some of the best cancer surgeons in the world and it would have taken only a couple calls to get her an appointment.

"I am having it next week," she said, not missing a beat. "The surgeon's schedule was pretty open. I like him and the radiologist referred me."

Not wanting to slow the process, I acquiesced. We hung up and I remember turning on the news to try to calm myself down just in time to catch an anchor teasing the next story: "Tampa surgeon removes wrong leg. Details after the break!" I turned the TV off. Einstein theorized that time can be distorted and waiting for biopsy results proves it—every minute becomes an hour.

Finally, her appointment passed and she called. "It was negative. I am all clear!" she said. I breathed a huge sigh of relief and as we chatted, I happened to bring up the story I had seen of the surgeon who had removed the wrong leg.

"By the way, Mom, what was the name of your surgeon?" I asked. You guessed it—it was the poor guy who had taken off a patient's healthy leg. With a son who could have gotten her to the finest surgeon in the world, my mother let herself be stuck with a man whose name would become synonymous with medical error. No wonder he had room in his schedule!

Luckily my mother's choice not to use choice had no repercussions. But allowing yourself to fall into substandard care doesn't always end well. One of the most common reasons patients don't get the best care for them is because their insurance doesn't cover it. Again, and this is hugely important: your insurance will determine your care. This means that getting the best care starts with choosing the best plan.

This is why I'm going to suggest something radical here: let the care you need determine what insurance you choose. Really, instead of slipping into whatever insurance plan is easiest, do your homework to figure out what care you need—the best doctors, specialists, and facilities for you and your family—and then pick the plan that covers these components. This flips the traditional workflow of insurance and healthcare on its ear. Most people will end up in an insurance plan and then look around within the plan to see which doctors, specialists, and facilities are covered. I'm telling you to do something radically different: choose your doctors, specialists, and facilities first. Then, no matter what your insurance options are, sort through these options to figure out which plans cover the things you need.

Of course, there are some situations in which you *have* to pick your plan first. If your finances dictate a certain plan, you may have no choice. Or expensive/specific medications may limit your insurance options. Or specialty services such as mental healthcare may make your choice of insurance plans for you. But if you can—if there are two or more possible options for you—*pick your team first and your insurance plan second.*

Now that you know the best workflow for picking health insurance, let's get into the nitty-gritty of how to do it. Sports writer Matt Bowen describes seven factors that free agents should consider when choosing which NFL team to sign with—money, location, taxes, playing for a winner, coaching familiarity, the playbook, and family life—and the idea is the same when choosing health insurance. A complex mix of factors can help you make the best decision for you.

One important factor is your primary care physician. If you have a relationship with your doctor, it would be a shame to pick an insurance plan that forces you to switch. Great doctors, like great coaches, connect beyond medicine, understanding the impact they can have on patients' lives.

For example, my father has had diabetes for 60 years. I think "insulin reaction" were practically my first words. The other day, I was talking to him on the phone and it was obvious from his slurred speech that his blood sugar was low. At first I was stern: "Dad, go get some orange juice now!" He ignored me, rambling incoherently. Then I tried to be nicer: "Dad, you know your sugar is low, don't even check it, just get a candy bar or your glucose tablets." It didn't work. He was attempting to check his sugar and finally was able to tell me the number, 33, which is dangerously low. Then he went silent on me. I yelled "Dad! Dad! Dad! Talk to me!" But there was only silence. I never felt more powerless. Was he passed out? Was he going to die on the phone with me? I hung up to call his wife, my stepmother, and she said she would be home from the store in minutes. Just before dialing 911, I called Dad back and, miraculously, he answered. I coaxed him into drinking orange juice and he began to improve.

If it weren't for his relationship with his endocrinologist, this close call could have been much worse. My dad's doctor knows he can be a strong-headed patient. To hedge against Dad's goal to keep his sugar as low as possible, his endocrinologist has reduced his insulin, leaving his blood sugar a little on the high side. This leaves him a bigger cushion on the low side. His doctor also knows that my dad sometimes takes insulin before his appointments just because he's the kind of patient who wants to get the best score on his blood test. This means that even if a test comes back perfect in the office, it might not be a true representation of my dad's blood sugar at home. My dad's doctor knows these things—he knows my dad—and so he's able to adjust my dad's care in a way no one else could. If you have a good specialist or PCP, that relationship, knowledge, and connection can be invaluable.

A second important factor when picking your health insurance is whether you or your loved ones will need specialty care. If you or a loved one on your plan has specific needs including mental health, substance abuse, chronic medical conditions, specialized therapy needs, or other special services, this could force you to pick a plan that covers care for these conditions. If your condition is complex and severe, having access to top-notch facilities and specialists becomes important (for example, access to a National Cancer Institute-designated cancer center). If your condition is chronic, like heart disease, diabetes, or arthritis, or if you have a mix of conditions, then access to an excellent primary care physician moves to the top of the priority list.

Third, ask how easy it will be to access the care you need. Some plans (especially HMOs) require a referral from your PCP in order to see a specialist. This makes your PCP a so-called "gatekeeper" that you will have to go through before you can see a specialist. But if your condition requires frequent specialist care, it can be cumbersome to go through your PCP when you know it's just a hoop to jump through on the way to the care you really need. For example, someone with diabetes may end up using their endocrinologist like a primary care physician to manage all aspects of their condition. The same is true of dialysis patients and patients with HIV. If you will be using your specialist like a primary care physician, it's worth looking into plans that offer direct access.

Then think about other factors that will affect your decision. Do you travel? If so, you will want a plan that allows you the flexibility to use doctors in other locations. Is money not a major issue? You will want a plan that allows you to choose the very best. In all of these special cases, start by choosing your team first—determine what care you want and then choose the plan that allows access.

So the crux of choosing health insurance becomes less about sorting through plans and more about sorting through your healthcare options. Who is the best doctor and who are the best specialists? It can be difficult to tell. Maybe that's why so many people end up with "good enough" care, settling for whatever doctor is closest or whichever specialist happens to be their referral. The next section of this chapter will lead you through the process of evaluating the people who deliver your care. This can be a cumbersome procedure, but the good news is that you shouldn't have to do it very often. Use the following steps to choose the doctors who will manage your health for years to come.

## Picking a Doctor

### GENERAL CHARACTERISTICS

1. **Gender:** Do you have a preference for your PCP's or specialist's gender? Some plans may have only a few options in your area and so it's worth asking whether the providers you will be allowed to see match this preference.

2. **Language and culture:** This can be very important if you or your family don't speak English.

3. **Level of experience or age:** Do you prefer a seasoned doctor or someone who is right out of training? In general, the more complicated or rare your medical problems, the more experience matters.

4. **Who calls the plays?** Do you want to decide your care or do you want a doctor to make your decisions for you? When evaluating doctors, ask about their approach to shared decision-making.

5. **Do they have another specialty?** Some PCPs have training or interest in certain conditions. Likewise, a specialist may be willing to manage a patient's routine care, like a PCP.

6. **What is their approach to wellness?** Does the provider prioritize nutrition, lifestyle choices, and other preventative care?

7. **What is their stance on integrating alternative medicines and spirituality in your care?** This can be very important for anyone who has strong feelings about including these in a more holistic approach.

8. **Doctors who teach:** When you see a doctor at an academic medical center you may have a preeminent doctor managing your care, but may be seen first by doctors in training.

9. **Location and convenience:** It may be important to balance your need for specialty care against your need for convenience. This encompasses how easy it is to get to the treatment location and also the efficiency of the office. Is the doctor always running behind? Is it because

he or she is willing to spend more time with their patients?

10. **Advance Nurse Practitioners or Physician Assistants:** Some doctors use these professionals as key members of their team. I have family members who rarely if ever see the doctor, and they love it. I have others who insist on seeing their doctor every time. It is important to know the standard operating procedure of the doctor you are considering.

11. **Hospital care:** If your PCP works in a hospital, he or she may be able to manage your care when hospital visits are needed. If your PCP doesn't work in a hospital setting, he or she may turn your care over to a "hospitalist" to manage your hospital care. In that case, the hospitalist becomes your interim head coach, the doctor who over-sees a patient's care in the hospital before handing this role back to a patient's PCP when he/she is discharged. Of course, the consideration of whether your PCP has hospital privileges or will need to hand off to a hospitalist is more important for patients who have to go to the hospital often.

## RED FLAGS

1. Is the doctor board certified and if not, why not?
2. Is the doctor on the national practitioner database for a violation that was reported?
3. Has the provider been sanctioned by the state medical board?
4. Has the doctor been the subject of malpractice claims?
5. Has the doctor lost hospital privileges currently or in the past?

6. Is he or she in databases for Medicare fraud or excessive testing, prescribing, or billing?

## WEBSITE INFORMATION

1. Where did he/she go to medical school?
2. Where did he/she do their residency or fellowship?
3. How long has he/she been in practice?
4. What is the tone of the rules and instructions?
5. What are their channels of communication including phone, email, text, patient portal, and so forth?
6. How many other doctors and providers are in the practice?
7. Is this doctor in fact an MD, or is this person an Advanced Nurse Practitioner or other type of provider? If other than an MD, does this person have oversight from a physician?
8. Go to Healthfinder.gov for great tips on how to find your best doctor/coach!

## REVIEWS

Reviews and patient testimonies on a provider's website might be cherry-picked to include only the good ones. Instead, evaluate the reviews you find on HealthGrades.com or Angie's List. *Consumer Reports* also collects doctor ratings. Keep in mind that one or two disgruntled patients may be very vocal, but that a few bad reviews may not be an accurate reflection of the doctor or practice.

## Evaluating a Doctor: Call and Visit

Once your list is narrowed to a few promising options, it's time for the real test: calling the office and then a visit. When you call the office, have your questions ready. If you are considering a practice, let the receptionist know and ask if you can talk to the practice manager. In addition to answers to your questions, *how* they answer is telling. Is the office friendly, attentive, and helpful? Finally, you never really know if a doctor or practice will be a good match until you try it out. I have had many patients schedule a first appointment just to meet me and evaluate my practice. Your first visit will be the best indicator of whether you made the right choice. When I spoke with NFL quarterback Donovan McNabb about choosing coaches, he said, "All coaches have their style but the message is the same." Make sure a doctor's style is a match for you!

That said, choice may not be easy. In the summer of 2015, Health Affairs "secret shoppers" conducted a survey of 743 PCPs from five of California's nineteen insurance marketplace-pricing regions. In fewer than 30 percent of cases consumers were able to schedule an appointment with their first choice of provider. In part, this was due to doctors being listed as providers of certain insurances but not, in fact, taking that insurance. In other cases, many good doctors were simply not taking new patients. If your first attempts at picking a doctor aren't successful, try and try again! Establishing yourself as the patient of a doctor you trust can take time but is an essential step toward receiving the care you need.

Only once you've picked a doctor is it time to wade into the wild world of picking an insurance plan.

# CHAPTER 3:
## "INSECURANCE"

Timothy was the kind of patient you never forget—the father we strive to be. After months of nagging back pain, his wife had dragged him to her doctor at their small community clinic. It was more than a slipped disc and now Timothy had been transferred to my care in the hospital Intensive Care Unit (ICU). Surrounded by his loving wife and children, all eyes were on me as I opened the door to his room. I had read his chart and they saw the concern on my face. I tried to explain what "multi-lobular mass" and "encapsulating the renal artery" meant. They got the gist: things were not good.

Not all masses are cancer—it could have been an infection or some strange immune disease—and so at his prior hospital a surgeon had attempted a biopsy. Unfortunately, Timothy's mass was so deep in his abdomen and was so enmeshed with major arteries that the surgeon wasn't able to get the sample we needed. It was what surgeons in their dark humor call an "open and shut case"—they open up a patient, can't do anything, and so close the patient back up. Our attempt at diagnosis was back to square one.

After I explained the predicament to Timothy's family, I began to search for someone who might again attempt to biopsy his mass with needles or surgery…or, heck, I would have settled for X-ray vision at that point.

Unfortunately, during this time the mass continued its corporal coup, turning his organs against him. Time was running out. The mass was growing and Timothy's kidneys began to shut down. His blood pressure slid lower by the day. I brought in many specialists to no avail, all saying they couldn't fight an unknown enemy and that without a diagnosis they would be shooting in the dark. After the first failed attempt, no surgeon in our system would touch him with a 10-foot scalpel. And there remained the nagging fear that the mass may not be cancer—if you blast an infection with chemotherapy or steroids, you just feed the beast. Likewise, even assuming the mass was cancer, choosing the wrong cancer-fighting cocktail would only speed his death.

In desperation, I attempted to transfer Timothy to a larger academic medical center three hours away. And after reviewing his films and data, a surgeon at the center was willing to have another shot at biopsy. I was elated! His family literally jumped with jubilation at the news. Timothy had one last chance.

That's when we heard from his insurance company.

Timothy had spent so many days in the hospital that his bare-bones insurance plan had run out. He had exceeded his annual limit. Timothy had health insurance…but not enough. The ICU nurse at the academic medical center gave me the bad news: they would not accept Timothy's transfer unless the family sent a check for $50,000 up front! The family didn't have anywhere near that kind of money. Who does?

I dreaded entering Timothy's room that day, knowing that his fate had been written years ago when he signed up for subpar insurance in some human resources office. Disgusted but obligated to inform the family, I watched hope drain from their faces. "You can't be serious!" his daughter shouted. After the shock, they actually went about searching among their family and friends for the cash. Never getting near the goal, Timothy died a week later.

Insurance was around long before money. In the early days of human society, insurance was essentially an agreement to help out when disaster like a collapsed hut or illness or crop failure struck. You "paid" your effort into the system and then when you needed it, could recoup aid in return. You can even think of sharing food as a kind of insurance: a successful hunter "paid" meat to the insurance co-op for the privilege of being allowed to share a meal on days his arrows missed their mark. Sharing resources and aid decreased risk and increased security in times when food, clothes, shelter and survival were far from guaranteed.

As civilization started using money, so did insurance. Now rather than having to contribute food or work or assistance to an insurance co-op, people could represent all these things with money and pay it to the system instead. The first formalized health insurance in the United States was a hospital prepayment plan, started in the 1920s. After World War II, as the country reinvented itself as a nation of industrialized workers, insurance became linked with employment.

Of course, that's exactly how it worked and since the 1920s the United States has been coasting on the tracks of a perfectly oiled health insurance machine with no gaps, flaws, or friction points.

Okay, maybe that's not quite true. In 1900 the average person spent $5 annually on healthcare, about $130 in today's dollars. According to the National Council of State Legislatures, in 2012 the average American paid $951 for health insurance premiums alone, not to mention the out-of-pocket spending I call "OOPs!" (much more on that later). Of course, a major culprit of the rising cost of health insurance is the rising cost of healthcare. Healthcare costs have risen every year since data has been kept (except for a brief stint in the late 1990s when managed care placed price above quality), with economists generally divided along political lines in their opinions of what drives the pace of this growth.

Believe me, I know many doctors long for the days before the money. Couldn't we just go back to insurance collectives in which I help raise your barn and you help rebuild mine after a fire?

Insurance isn't alone in this problem of spiraling costs in which money can trump the needs of the very people it's supposed to protect. The same has happened in football. As you've seen, the NFL is a team of teams and the whole system is built on sharing. Only, here's a big difference between the NFL and healthcare: the NFL is built to share revenue and healthcare is built to share costs. The NFL wants to maximize revenue and healthcare seeks to reduce cost. Despite being different levers, both systems of sharing are meant to have the same effect on the bottom line: money is squeezed toward the middle. Rich teams share profits to make sure that poor teams are competitive and healthy patients pay into insurance systems so that sick patients can afford care. And, unfortunately, neither system completely evens out the gap between rich and poor—the New England Patriots are still able to spend more on their roster than the Jacksonville Jaguars and across diseases, poor patients still have worse outcomes than wealthier ones. Despite these systems designed to share costs, the rich prosper and the poor can be left behind.

Ironically, there are about 32 major American insurance companies, the same as the number of NFL owners. And like NFL owners drafting players, most Americans are drafted onto their insurance teams. The vast majority of Americans don't choose health insurance—it chooses them. Like the NFL draft, you sit in an auditorium waiting for your name to be called before walking to the front to claim the jersey and the hat of the insurance team that becomes your owner.

According to the Kaiser Family Foundation's Employer Health Benefit Survey, 81 percent of companies with more than 200 employees are self-insured. This means that just like the running back who always dreamed of playing for his sunny hometown team but ends up drafted into a Rust Belt franchise where athletes play on "tundra" rather than "turf," instead of choosing your insurance team, you're more likely to end up drafted onto your employer's team of choice.

And like NFL teams, not all health insurance companies are created equal. The second you complete a hospital intake, you are labeled by your team as if your insurance card is your jersey. You can almost hear the office staff saying, "He is Blue Cross. She is that pain-in-the-neck local plan...I hate them." The problem is not just that quality varies in health insurance, meaning that some patients play for more respected teams than others. The problem is that *you have very little choice what team you play for.* See, you've heard the phrase money talks, but in this case your money is mute. Because you don't really choose who gets your insurance premiums, the company doesn't have to please you. The American healthcare system now costs about $3 trillion dollars (that's trillion with a "T") per year and the bad news is, to use language from the previous chapter, that as the costs for the team have risen, so have the costs for the "me." Americans' out-of-pocket spending is up 73 percent just since 1996. Premiums have increased even more, rising 147 percent. One-in-five Americans cannot afford some aspect of their medical care.

Think about it like paying for a dinner bill while on a business trip. Imagine you order a reasonable meal and your company picks up the tab. Great! No out-of-pocket costs for you. That was the early days of healthcare: we consumed a reasonable amount of healthcare and our employers basically paid the entire tab. Well, we learned that when someone else is picking up the tab, we might as well get the lobster! How many times do you think you could order lobster on your employer's ticket before your employer decided to start passing along some of the cost to you? That's what happened in the 1970s and 1980s—with someone else picking up the bill, patients were blind to cost, healthcare costs went up, and now employers and insurance companies are asking you to chip in for the lobster.

Now, it seems reasonable to believe that if you're asked to pay for part of your meal, you might think twice about ordering something extravagant. But here's where the analogy breaks down: We don't consume healthcare the way we consume meals. When it comes to health, we make some strange decisions. For example, some people decide to keep ordering the lobster, no matter what it costs; some people *need* the lobster and don't have any choice; then some people decide that if they're asked to share some of the cost, they'll skip the meal altogether...until they discover they're starving and the meal costs five times as much. Still others look at the menu and just make bad

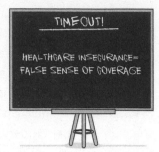

choices, overspending on things that are inconsequential and underspending on things that could make a dramatic difference. Think about this in terms of your own health insurance and healthcare: are you eating the lobster? Are you skipping the meal? One decision comes with cost and the other comes with risk, representing a major tradeoff seen in so much of our health insurance system.

Certainly, the Affordable Care Act (ACA) increased the number of insured Americans but it didn't do much for Americans caught in what I call the "OOPs" gap—the people who have insurance but are caught unaware by out-of-pocket expenses, as in "OOPs you owe $8,000 dollars!" Today, like Timothy whose insurance turned down his chance to be diagnosed and thus treated for what was probably renal cancer, one in five patients have been forced to abandon or postpone treatment because they cannot afford it.

These "OOPs-es!" are written into your 60-page health insurance policy in fine-print judicial jargon that might as well be medieval Russian. The ACA has tried to simplify and standardize these documents and open the process of shopping for insurance. (That is, if you are a rare free agent able to take advantage of this marketplace and not drafted onto a team not of your choosing—much more on this later.) The law also did away with some of the limits that took Timothy's last chance, with the "patient protection" part of the act ensuring Timothy was at least afforded the opportunity to receive what could have been a life-saving diagnosis.

No law, however, can escape the whack-a-mole nature of sharing risk in the healthcare game—take away restrictions and price pops up; leave the price restrictions in place and quality problems pop up. You can't hit one without raising the other. The ACA's answer was to encourage healthy people to join the team.

It was a tough sell. Why would a healthy person choose to overpay for insurance they don't expect to need? The inability to tempt healthy people into the system meant that insurers lost money. Aetna and United Healthcare dropped out. In addition to defections, according to an 18-state analysis by McKinsey & Company, the composition of plans changed to HMOs or others that offered access to similarly restricted networks.

Insurers were left with a devil's choice: Increase premiums or increase OOPs. They are doing both. Employers are only middlemen, passing along the higher cost of insurance plans to their employees. Take the time to look at your most recent benefits statement. Chances are your company is asking you to pay more if not all of your premium, and your deductible, co-pays, and co-insurance have all gone up. According to Drew Altman, President and CEO of the Kaiser Family Foundation, employees are now paying nearly one-third or an average of $5,277 of their family premiums, and deductibles for 80 percent of employees average $1,500 with employees at smaller companies carrying an average $2,100 deductible. As painful as it is to look, the alternative is the OOPs! being caught by surprise when something you expect to be covered is suddenly not.

If the ACA's answer to paying out more than it brings in was to raise premiums (while trying to offset these increases with subsidies for the most vulnerable), another approach is to raise OOPs. Again, the decision of whether to increase premiums or increase OOPs spills over into politics, which is something I'm trying *very hard* not to do in this book. Again, Democrats generally prefer raising premiums with the pain offset by subsidies, while Republicans generally favor raising OOPs while encouraging people to put aside money for these OOPs in tax-advantaged HSAs. The gist is that it's a challenge on both sides of the political aisle.

The other day, I was reading the book *The Game Before the Money: Voices of the Men Who Built the NFL*, by Jackson Michael, and it reminded me of a time in healthcare "before the money." When I went to medical school it was not only impolite but also unethical to allow money into medical care. We were taught to do what our patients needed at any cost. Our focus was on quality. We were all out to dinner at the best restaurant in town on our employer's dime. Now, times have changed, the bill is in our own pockets, and we can't pay. Until you win the lottery, or insurance, healthcare, and government find a way to fix the system, we'll all be scrubbing plates in the kitchen to work off our meal.

Feeling more secure yet?

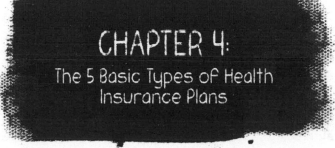

# CHAPTER 4:
## The 5 Basic Types of Health Insurance Plans

A health insurance "plan" seems like an oxymoron—don't we have health insurance specifically for those *unplanned* times? Over time, health insurance has evolved from a way to protect against catastrophic accidents and illnesses to the way we pay for most of our healthcare. By the 1990s, employers paid our premiums, insurance companies paid for our treatments, and we bought healthcare like a kid with his parent's credit card. This resulted in the backlash known as managed care, in which plans managed doctors who managed your care and, unfortunately, who prioritized cost savings over the quality of care.

During this time, I worked in a Medicare HMO where we were paid a dollar amount per patient per month, whether or not we saw the patient. Sounds reasonable, right? The problem is that over time when I tried to refer these managed care patients to my specialist partners they suddenly had no empty slots. Why fill those slots with patients to earn a minimal monthly fee when full-paying patients were waiting to be seen?

Health insurance evolved in the 1990s and is evolving again dramatically today. The thing to keep in mind is that every plan has pros and cons—but by knowing these plans you can maximize the pros and minimize the cons *for your specific situation*. Not every person will be best served by an HMO. Not everyone fits in Medicare Advantage. And not everyone needs a high-premium private plan. As you descend into this jungle of health insurance acronyms, think about the tradeoffs between premiums and out-of-pocket costs, ease and freedom, basic care and specialty care, and maybe most importantly, known costs and the costs associated with risk. We'll get into the specifics of choosing insurance in later chapters. For now, try to get a flavor for these basic kinds of health insurance plans.

## Health Maintenance Organization (HMO)

This is the most common kind of health insurance, covering 30 percent of insured Americans and representing the majority of plans offered in marketplaces. HMOs are usually inexpensive and easy to manage, including the lowest out-of-pocket expenses. The drawback is that your care is restricted to primary care providers and specialists within the HMO organization. Except for emergency care, expect to pay *way* more to see an out-of-network provider. If you expect to require specialty care, make sure your HMO includes the specialists or specialty hospitals you need (this can be especially important for cancer patients). As long as your HMO (or EPO, see the following) includes the specialists and facilities you need, your experience with the HMO can be easy and productive. Remember that when you choose an HMO you are giving up freedom for lower cost. You are required to have a PCP and will need his or her approval to see most specialists. HMOs tend to be very local and may not work well when you're out of your home region. If you expect to seek most of your care locally and within one system, an HMO can be easy and your best value.

## Exclusive Provider Organization (EPO)

An EPO is like an HMO made up of independent doctors. It's a group of independent or private providers who have agreed to provide care under an insurance agreement. This makes an EPO like a hybrid of an HMO and a PPO in that you restrict yourself to a defined care network, and in return pay less for care within this network. In most EPOs you can see specialists without first getting a referral from your PCP, making this a good choice for someone who needs frequent specialty care— rather than going through the gatekeeper of your PCP every time, an EPO usually lets you skip this step and head straight for the specialist.

## Preferred Provider Organization (PPO)

A PPO is less restrictive than an HMO or EPO, but more choice usually comes with more cost and, potentially, more head-aches. As its name implies, some providers are "preferred" but you can choose to go elsewhere, usually without the dramatic penalties of an HMO or EPO. Many PPOs don't require that you have a primary care physician, allowing you to schedule directly with a specialist, if needed.

## High Deductible Health Plan (HDHP)

Are you young, healthy, or don't get sick much? It can be tempting to buy a low-cost HDHP, also known as a *catastrophic coverage plan*. However, these cheap plans can have limited coverage and come with the most risk for a big bill. Expect to pay many of your expenses out-of-pocket. Many people bundle an HDHP with a Health Savings Account (HSA) to pay these out-of-pocket expenses with pre-tax dollars. In fact, in order to have an HSA, you specifically must have an HDP and pairing these two—HDP with HSA—has grown in popularity. However, be aware that with HSA plans, you might not be able to have basic visits and care covered pre-deductible as you can with some other plans. According to Health and Human Services data, in 2010, 25.3 percent of privately insured patients were on HDPs, jumping to 36.7 percent in 2015. At the same time, the percentage of people with HSAs went from 7.7 to 13.3 percent. In my mind, the major danger of an HDP is the chance that you will skimp on vital care. If you're paying out-of-pocket, will you choose to skip important medications or treatments?

## Point of Service (POS)

These plans combine an HMO's requirement to start your services with a designated primary care physician, but then like a PPO allow you to go out-of-network to receive specialty care. Again, in healthcare you tend to pay for choice—POS has more choice than HMO and is usually more expensive; POS has less choice and is usually less expensive than PPO.

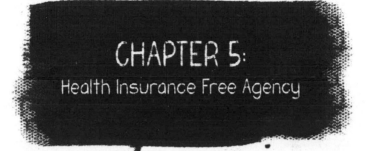

# CHAPTER 5:
## Health Insurance Free Agency

In the fall of 1969, MLB Golden Glove winner Curtis Flood learned from reporters that he was going to be traded to the Philadelphia Phillies from his team, the St. Louis Cardinals. The Phillies were terrible at the time, and Flood refused to be traded. He wrote a letter to the commissioner of baseball asking to be allowed to join another team or become a free agent. Here is part of that letter:

> After twelve years in the major leagues, I do not feel I am a piece of property to be bought and sold irrespective of my wishes. I believe that any system which produces that result violates my basic rights as a citizen and is inconsistent with the laws of the United States and of the several States...
>
> I have received a contract offer from the Philadelphia club, but I believe I have the right to consider offers from other clubs before making any decision. I, therefore, request that you make known to all Major League clubs

my feelings in this matter, and advise them of my availability for the 1970 season.

His team and the commissioner denied his request and,
with the support of the Players' Union, Flood decided to sue.
The case eventually made its way to the United States Supreme
Court as Flood vs. Kuhn. Flood lost, with the high court ruling
that Major League Baseball was a sport and not a business
and so a different calculation of Flood's rights applied. But
Flood had laid the groundwork and in 1975 the Supreme Court
reversed its decision, opening the era of baseball free agency
and paving the way for free agency in other leagues.

By 1992 the NFL was ready for its own test of free agency.
That year, the Philadelphia Eagle's Reggie White (initially a
standout in the USFL) was the best player in the NFL. He was
also a role model off the field, the "Minister of Defense" on
Sundays and in the off season, literally a minister at his church.
Philadelphia fans loved him—and these were the people who
famously threw snowballs at Santa Claus! That spring Reggie
White was on the cover of *Sports Illustrated* with the caption,
"What Jersey will he wear?" Green Bay, Washington, and the
Forty-Niners all bid to steal him away.

Until Reggie White, players generally spent their careers
with one team. Now players had the power of choice—the
power to choose from the teams that wanted them. Reggie
White did his homework, visiting these teams. It was a sharp
role reversal, the player evaluating teams instead of teams
evaluating the player. Reggie White asked what the coaches
were like, what sort of system their defenses played, and what
that would mean for him. He factored in the location, the
weather, the distance from family, and the stadium. And of

course, since football is truly both a sport and a business, he took into account the money. He also took into account the things these organizations could offer that were unique to his individual needs.

That spring, in a tearful news conference, Reggie White said goodbye to Philadelphia fans. The next season, he played for Green Bay, which had offered to pay for a plane to fly him to Milwaukee to preach to troubled youth. More so than money or glory, Reggie White did his research and chose his team based on how well it fit him as a person.

The relevance of these stories is that healthcare, like sports leagues, is transitioning toward a model that increasingly includes free agency. Before sports free agency, team owners had all the power and players were drafted and stayed with that team unless they were traded, cut or retired. Falcons executive Rich McKay explained that even after free agency, the salary cap hoped to keep balance between teams, putting the league first. Before the Affordable Care Act, insurers had all the power and patients had little choice in their plan and could be cut or dropped from their health insurance at any time (typically if they were costing the insurer too much money). The ACA enacted rules against ruthless practices like denying coverage for people with preexisting conditions or selling blocks of patients to other companies. However, these changes came with a price. For example, forcing insurance companies to accept any patient, with premium increases only for age and smoking, means that some healthy people will pay higher premiums to make up for unhealthy people on the plan needing more care.

Like sports, the transition toward free agency isn't smooth. Some pioneering consumers are testing their choices, while others don't even realize a choice exists. This time in health-care reminds me of the summer I told my dad I didn't want to play baseball anymore. I only spent snippets of summers with my dad in Indiana and during those visits we quickly fell into a father-son cadence: after work he would change out of his Mr. Rogers shirt and tie and we would have our nightly catch. Unfortunately, my dad had a Nolan Ryan arm. The firecracker *pop* of his throws hitting my glove sent birds scattering from trees and the searing shock reverberated through my hand. For him, this was pure joy. For me...it just *hurt*. And back home in central Pennsylvania, I had fallen in love with football, which was becoming a year-round commitment.

From inside the "system" of these summer visits, it didn't seem like I had a choice. It was my job to be on the receiving end of my dad's 70 mph fastballs even though it hurt my hand and, really, I had already slid from the game. The thing is, I *did* have a choice. It just took initiative to find it and courage to enforce it. We could still have our nightly catch, but with a football instead of a rock-hard projectile that left my left palm bruised.

In healthcare, you have choices too. And just like making the difficult decision to tell my dad I was done with baseball, it can take initiative to discover that you *have* choice and courage to *use* it. Unfortunately, even once we discover we *have* choice, many people don't know what to do with it. For example, a study of 50,000 employees by the National Bureau of Economic Research found that when presented with four insurance benefit plans, 65 percent failed to choose the option that would have been best for them. These poor choices cost each employee another $373 per year in unnecessary spending. Even with some training another study demonstrated that patients make many mistakes in figuring out their out-of-pocket costs, or OOPs, for procedures and prescriptions.

The choices that let you find your best healthcare fit are some of the most important choices you will ever make, and yet statistics show you are ill equipped to make them. This isn't your fault! It is the system. Healthcare in the United States has become so complex and convoluted that doctors can't navigate it themselves. Many patients stop trying, preferring instead to stumble blindly into whatever plan seems easiest. With that attitude, Curtis Flood would have been traded to the then-dismal Philadelphia Phillies. Reggie White might have ended up with the organization that forked over the most cash, without respecting him as a person. And you could end up paying hundreds or thousands of dollars more for health insurance and healthcare that does less to meet your individual needs.

What this means is that the new era of healthcare free agency comes with opportunity, but it also comes with danger. Now that you have choice, you also have the ability to make the *wrong* choice. Unless you put your foot down, you end up on a default health insurance plan with a default primary care physician with backup at a default hospital. With this attitude, John Elway would have ended up playing for the Colts. The team used the first pick in the famous 1983 draft to secure Elway as their quarterback of the future. But Elway didn't want to play for the Colts. In college, he had been a baseball star as well as a football star and with the Yankees offering him a spot on the farm team, Elway told the Colts that instead of moving to Indianapolis, he would just go play baseball instead (in a kind of ironic reversal of my own decision with my dad). Before Elway, it was pretty much a done deal that football players would play for the team that drafted them. That was how the system worked. But Elway discovered that he had choice and then enforced it. Not wanting to lose the value of their first-round pick, the Colts traded Elway to Denver and the rest is history.

For you, the first step is to recognize when you are a free agent. The distinction is rarely clear; usually you will have some choice within the constraints of a system. In the following chapters, we'll look at some of these constraints—maybe your finances mean that you will be drafted onto one of the government-run insurance programs like Medicaid or CHIP; maybe you will have choices restricted by the plans offered by your employer; or maybe you will be an undrafted free agent, released to choose your plan on the exchanges or whatever free-market system replaces them.

These citizens who use the federal health insurance exchanges are the real free agents. And patient choice may be healthcare's secret weapon in the value crisis. Why? Give patients choice, information, and some skin in the game and they will make right choices and in doing, generally end up with the care they need while avoiding paying for care they do not. When patients wield this power of choice, they force healthcare teams to innovate and compete to win them over, creating more value. However, choice without enough transparency to really know how to weigh the options is just chance. And, in fact, both sides of the political aisle are pushing for greater transparency and comparability, some-thing I call "comparency." Republican plans tend to pair this comparency with more choice, for example with ideas like paying Medicare benefits in lump sums of cash and depending on consumers to choose how and if to spend the benefit on healthcare. Democratic plans tend to pair comparency with benefits, allowing consumers choice among plans, but not the choice to take cash instead of benefits and opt out completely.

The fact is that no matter the political climate, if you sit by the phone on draft day and don't get a call, you now have options—you have more right and more ability to demand to join a team. In all these situations, the first step is to recognize these choices and then find the courage to use them. When do you have the choice and thus the power? Can you choose your plan, your doctor, your hospital, your covered medications? And what is the cost of this choice? By asking yourself these questions, you can be Curtis Flood, John Elway, and Reggie White, secure with the health insurance team that fits your needs.

# CHAPTER 6:
## Drafted - Government-Run Insurance Programs

Of all the tragic consequences of poverty, lack of access to healthcare could be the most egregious. America is the only world power that does not make affordable healthcare available to all its citizens. The Affordable Care Act hoped to change that by drafting poor patients into Medicaid. Less restrictive federal Medicaid criteria led to a dramatic expansion, with more than 15 million Americans joining the team. In the future, the mechanics of offering affordable care to financially disadvantaged populations may change, but now that the genie of near-universal care is out of the bottle, it will be extremely difficult to put back in.

Of course, expanding any healthcare program costs money. Traditionally, the federal government has paid 60 percent and states pay 40 percent of Medicaid costs. When the ACA expanded Medicaid, it promised to pay 90 percent of the new costs (paying 100 percent during a break-in period). States were skeptical of this promise, in part because the federal government would only be paying for *expansion*—to cover new Medicaid patients who weren't eligible under the old rules. However, states knew that in addition to newly eligible enrollees, due to the marketing push they would see new signups from people who were previously eligible but hadn't been aware of the program or hadn't taken advantage of it before (states dubbed this the "woodwork effect"). The federal government would only give their standard 60 percent toward covering these previously eligible new enrollees. As you know, the bottom line was that many states were displeased.

How would the federal government compel states to make this expansion? They gave states a non-choice option: expand Medicaid and take all the offered federal dollars or don't expand Medicaid and lose all federal funds for the program. But it turned out that the states *did* have a choice: 30 states sued the federal government to throw out the law because of the individual mandate and the fact that they were being coerced into expanding Medicaid.

The rest is history. Chief Justice John Roberts saved the law, ruling in favor of the individual mandate but saying that the threat of withholding funds was too coercive and instead gave each state the option to expand Medicaid. Thirty states expanded, overwhelmingly along political lines (with exceptions like John Kasich, the Republican governor of Ohio, who expanded Medicaid against the wishes of his Republican-dominated state).

Here's what that means for you: If you are poor, even as rules change, there's a good chance you will be drafted into Medicaid (with some chance that in the future you could receive a lump sum distribution that you could use or not use for Medicaid). The only thing worse than being drafted by a team that isn't your top choice is not being drafted at all. Due to the inability of the ACA to ensure Medicaid expansion across all states, there are still millions of Americans who sit by the phone on draft day without ever getting a call. Because the law foresaw all states expanding Medicaid, federal subsidies for individuals buying plans on the exchange were not offered to those making less than 100 percent of FPL (who would receive Medicaid if expanded). Until rules are reworked under new administrations, this leaves the poorest of the poor in these non-expansion states stuck between a rock and a hard place, unable to qualify for a subsidy on bronze, silver, gold, or platinum plans and unable to receive Medicaid.

Now, Medicaid has its limitations but it is better than nothing. For those in need, it can be a lifesaving option. On the plus side, the program covers almost all of members' healthcare costs, with very little OOPs. That is, if you can find a doctor who accepts it. That's because Medicaid on average pays doctors less than Medicare and private health insurers. To encourage doctors to accept Medicaid patients, the ACA increased payments for the first two years of the program, but this incentive expired in 2014 and was not renewed. Some states picked up the slack and have kept this raise in place and more are likely to follow suit as it becomes clear that low Medicaid payouts limit the effectiveness of the program. In fact, I have been on the front line of this fight, visiting the offices of my state's representatives in Washington D.C. to implore them to keep what is called "parity" with Medicare-level payments, or in other words ensure that Medicaid pays just as much as Medicare.

Of course, there are doctors who choose to make less money so that they can serve underprivileged populations. As a PCP early in my career I told my group I would only take the job if I could work in a 100 percent Medicaid AIDS clinic one day a week. This meant a huge drop in my billing, to which they reluctantly agreed. However, trying to get some of my specialist partners to see those patients was like pulling teeth. They would see me in the hospital hallway and turn the other way, hoping not to be consulted. As a hospitalist, I have been fortunate enough to always take Medicaid patients. In fact, the company I work for has ensured that we doctors get paid the same amount whether we see a Medicaid or privately insured patient (similar to states choosing to create "parity" between Medicaid and Medicare). In other words, I've been very lucky— most of my work has been "insurance blind." Unfortunately, not every doctor can afford or agrees with this philosophy.

When I learned my personal doctor in Clearwater, Florida, does not take Medicaid, I decided to do a quick experiment—when I searched the Medicaid database for doctors in Clearwater who accept the insurance, about 120 popped up. Since I have practiced in this area for many years I know who are the top doctors from my point of view. I was happy to see that several doctors that I considered excellent were on the list but I didn't believe it. I called their offices to make sure. When I got through, I was told they didn't, in fact, take Medicaid. Many of the best PCPs were not on the list. Even fewer specialists accept Medicaid. To be fair, I didn't recognize all the names on the list and there may be some excellent options for Medicaid treatment in Clearwater, Florida…but from my extensive experience and also my quick search, options for Medicaid recipients are much more limited than for people with other insurances. If you have Medicaid, be prepared to make calls and do your homework to discover doctors you can have on your team.

The drafting doesn't stop there. Medicare, the government-run health insurance program most Americans contribute to through their paychecks, is basically your only option once you turn sixty-five. Sure, you can choose to pay out of pocket instead, but few have that kind of money. There is a glimmer of choice for the 30 percent of Americans who join Medicare Advantage health insurance (a kind of privatized Medicare option), but this choice, too, is evaporating. That's because big insurance companies keep buying on another. After this consolidation, many states and cities only have a few options, even in the world of Medicare Advantage. Who else is drafted onto their insurance? If you are an underprivileged child you are drafted into Children's Health Insurance Program or CHIP, which is a newer supplemental Medicaid just for kids. If you are in the military you are drafted into CHAMPUS, a plan limited to military hospitals. Veterans are drafted into the VA system with some limited ability to go to private non-VA doctors and hospitals.

Young adults who want to stay under their parents' insurance umbrella until 26 (as per the ACA) are drafted onto their parents' plan.

The bottom line is that it can be good to be drafted onto a government health insurance plan; at least these plans offer the option of insurance to people who might otherwise go uninsured. But with these plans, your choice is likely to be limited. Chances are you have no choice in the plan you are allowed to join, and then chances are your options are limited in how you use it. If you are drafted into Medicaid, Medicare,

CHIP, CHAMPUS, or any of these other programs, don't let your lack of options discourage you from exercising the choices that remain! You can still choose your PCP. You may still have choice in the hospitals and other facilities you use. In the future, these plans and your degree of choice within them is likely to change.

States are likely to be faced with tough choices too. Interestingly, states that were winners under the ACA may become losers as policies shift money away from the structures set up under the ACA. For example, the ACA promised to pay 90 percent of the costs for Medicaid expansion. Now these expansion states may be left holding the bill. And one possible future has the federal government offering block grants to all states, which may help people in non-expansion states buy private plans.

As the bedrock of government plans and your choices within these plans continues to shift, just make sure you know exactly what your options are. Then do your homework now, before you are sick, to discover which healthcare you can use. It's not worth waiting until you're sick or injured to start discovering the opportunities and limitations of your healthcare plan.

# CHAPTER 7:
## Restricted Free Agent
## Your Employer's Insurance Options

Sixty-five percent of Americans, about 165 million in all, get their health insurance through their employers, a system created in the period after WWII when employers started offering benefits as a way to court workers that were in incredibly high demand. Despite some healthcare experts and economists (for example Uwe Reinhardt and Ezekiel Emanuel) wishing it was not so, the system of health insurance paired with employment has been quite durable. In fact, 81 percent of companies with more than 200 employees act almost like their own insurance company, offering exclusive plans to their employees, with "real" insurance companies managing the details. This means that paying part or all of your health insurance premium is exactly the same as increasing your income, only, because your employer can pay your insurance with pre-tax dollars but would pay your salary in after-tax dollars, it's cheaper for your employer to increase your wage with benefits rather than with salary.

I'm not saying this is a bad thing. Actually, in most cases it's a win-win, with employees getting insurance that is effectively subsidized by their employer and businesses being able to "pay" their employees more without the raise costing them quite as much. Just as the ACA was meant to offer options for people who are not employed full-time, it is also meant to strengthen the requirement for businesses to offer insurance to employees who are. In part, this is accomplished by the employer mandate in which, starting in 2016, companies of a certain size have to offer affordable health insurance to 95 percent of their employees. The law also makes companies "auto-enroll" all new hires into their health insurance. Like it or not, you are being told to buy health insurance and companies are being told to offer it.

Here's the thing: A survey by Kaiser Health Insurance found that 52 percent of companies that employ more than 200 people offer only one plan. Thirty-nine percent offer two plans and 9 percent offer three or more. This means that if you have insurance through your employer, it's nearly 50/50 that you are drafted into your health insurance team with no choice in the matter—52 percent of people who work for large companies are not free agents at all! The reason is that by putting as many people as possible on a single plan, employers have more leverage to negotiate costs with insurance companies. Chances are that your employer saved you a couple bucks a month (and themselves more than a couple) by using the number of insurance enrollees to talk their insurer into a lower plan cost. But this savings comes at the cost of choice.

Let's start by taking a closer look at these 52 percent whose employers offer only one plan—take it or leave it! Of course, even if your employer offers only one choice for health insurance, you still have some choice in picking your doctor, hospital and other facilities, and specialists (within the network defined by your plan). And your choices within your employer's plan are likely to be more extensive than your choices in a government-run program like Medicaid.

You may also be able to encourage your business to adjust their plan. One point of leverage even for people whose employers offer only one plan is the ACA mandate that as of January 1, 2016, all companies with more than 50 employees must offer *affordable* and *minimum value* health insurance to all *full-time* employees or pay a penalty. "Affordable" means that the total cost of your individual health insurance must not exceed 9.66 percent of your household income. (A family plan can cost more.) "Minimum value" means that the plan must cover at least 60 percent of your cost of care. This is important: if your employer does not offer a plan that meets these minimum requirements, you may be eligible to go to Healthcare.gov and buy a plan of your choice, perhaps with subsidy. However, be aware that if you go this route (and don't qualify for Medicaid), your employer will be penalized.

You also have the choice to decline your employer's one health insurance plan, but for most of us, unless you have coverage through your spouse or partner's plan, it's not a very good choice. If you can't afford your employer's plan and buy an individual plan on a federal marketplace, your employer will be penalized (the ACA penalized $100/day). Under ACA rules, if you decline your employer's plan and choose to go without insurance completely, you would end up paying a tax penalty, not to mention accepting the risk of being without health insurance.

In other words, if your employer offers only one plan and you don't have another option from a spouse or partner, you're almost certainly stuck with it. You're drafted. And as long as your employer's plan meets designated requirements, your best strategy is probably to accept it and then work to find the best choices for you within the plan.

Now, some companies continue to offer a few or many health insurance options. In that case, you're like a restricted free agent: You can exercise choice within boundaries. If that's the case, choice can be as restricted as the pick between two plans offered by the same insurer ("single carrier"). Or your choice could let you shop across a number of insurers ("multi-carrier"). Still less restrictive, many companies are moving toward a model in which they offer employees a set amount of money to use toward insurance purchased through a private exchange. These private exchanges can't offer the subsidies of public ones, but an employer's "defined contribution" works in much the same way as a subsidy, paying a portion of your cost. According to Kaiser, 13 percent of companies have moved to this model, including Walgreens, Sears, and Darden Restaurants for full-time employee benefits; IBM, Time Warner, and General Electric for retiree benefits; and Target for part-time employees. Some estimates predict that 40 million Americans could get health insurance on private exchanges by 2018.

Employer-sponsored health insurance is the traditional way of doing things. Now there are many new options. But just because employer-sponsored insurance has been around almost 75 years doesn't mean it's outdated. Your employer may have negotiated a great deal with a strong insurance company, allowing you access to great care for much less than you would pay as an individual. Think about it: there is nothing wrong with being quarterback Terry Bradshaw, who spent his entire 14-year career with the Steelers and won four Super Bowls. That said, as healthcare and health insurance costs go up, employers are looking for ways to pass along some of these costs to their employees. In the future, this may make employer-sponsored insurance less attractive to employees. And at a certain point, you'd be better off taking an incentive from your employer to buy your own plan at Healthcare.gov.

The question is whether you're at that point now. If you're happy with your employer-sponsored plan, stick with it. If you're not, it's probably worth exploring your employer's other options first...if there *are* other options. And if you're fed up with your employer's rising premiums for falling care, consider seeing if your employer is just as fed up as you are. There's a chance that rather than keeping you on their health insurance team, your employer would be better off paying out your contract to let you enter the market as a free agent.

## A Note for Employers

In addition to exchanges for individuals buying health insurance, the ACA also created exchanges for small business owners evaluating health insurance options for their employees. Like Healthcare.gov, the website for the SHOP exchange had a delayed and bumpy launch. Originally, the marketplace was available only to businesses with 50 or fewer full-time employees offering insurance to all employees who work more than 30 hours per week. In addition, 70 percent of employees who are offered plans must accept them or enroll in individual insurance. Now some states are offering SHOP insurance to larger businesses and with different rules for which employees qualify.

Because the laws governing SHOP insurance vary from state to state and are constantly changing, if you are a small business owner, your best bet is probably to throw yourself on the mercy of the SHOP website, which will lead you through your current options. Like ACA individual insurance plans, SHOP offers subsidies to qualifying businesses. For example, if your small business has fewer than 25 full-time employees, you may be able to earn tax credits to offset half the cost of paying your employee's health insurance premiums. As any small business owner knows, offering health insurance can be a huge incentive to attract qualified candidates. And saving half the cost of this incentive is a significant break.

Of course, the rules governing SHOP, just like the rules governing the ACA, are up for debate. If there is any constant in healthcare, it is change. And one of these proposed changes dramatically decouples insurance from employment. This would be dramatic. And if there's anything our country can learn from the ACA is that dramatic changes to our healthcare system can come with pain. Therefore, while I expect changes like strengthened HSAs and perhaps even more lump-sum distributions from employers to employees, who will then be empowered to buy their own plans, I also expect the tried-and-true system of employer-sponsored health insurance to continue, no matter the political climate. The ACA and SHOP may be retired into the roles of coaches or broadcasters, but the fact is that small businesses should expect to continue navigating the rules of health insurance for their employees.

# CHAPTER 8:

## Undrafted Free Agents
## The ACA Marketplace

In 1928, three-month-old Dick Lane was abandoned in a dumpster in Austin, Texas. At first Ella Lane mistook his cries for the sound of a cat. To his good fortune, she investigated and when the cat turned out to be a baby, she ended up adopting and raising the child. Despite Dick Lane's accolades on the L.C. Anderson High School football team and while playing one year at a junior college, he joined the military at age nineteen. After four years, he got a job at an aircraft plant in Los Angeles. Then in 1952 he famously walked into the Los Angeles Rams headquarters and asked for a tryout. In his first play, Dick Lane made a powerful tackle on the team's best running back and went on to wreak havoc in the NFL. In his rookie season, he had 14 interceptions in a 12-game season, still a record today. In 1974, Dick "Night Train" Lane was inducted into the NFL Hall of Fame.

Undrafted does not mean that a team wouldn't be happy to have you.

As you've seen, most Americans are drafted onto their health insurance team through their jobs or through their life circumstances like Medicare (age) or Medicaid (income). Then there is a minority of employers that offer more than one plan making some of you restricted free agents. And then there are the undrafted, the Dick "Night Train" Lanes, left to fend for themselves. Ironically, like the incredible man himself, being an undrafted free agent can set you up to be the biggest winner.

The Affordable Care Act (ACA) is an oxymoron of mandates alongside freedom of choice, requiring that everyone buy health insurance (no choice) but then opening the possibilities for what insurance you buy (choice). In other words, the ACA is both a carrot and a stick—the individual mandate is the "stick," compelling Americans to buy insurance that is sometimes against their best interest, but benefits the team. (Supreme Court Justice Ruth Bader-Ginsberg famously called those that don't buy health insurance "free-riders," in that if they chose not to buy insurance and eventually end up needing health-care that they cannot afford, we all end up paying for it.) And the "carrot" is the increased choice offered in exchanges and marketplaces. Future systems may do away with the mandate, but the idea that insurance options should be available for all and that the government could compel our choices within these options is here to stay.

For example, in 2016, the tax penalty for refusal or inability to obtain the mandated health insurance was either $695 per adult plus $347.50 per child (up to $2,085 per family) or 2.5 percent of your total adjusted household income, whichever was greater. For 2017 and beyond, the plan of the ACA was to adjust the flat penalty for inflation to increase year-over-year. (Check Healthcare.gov current rules, especially as ACA laws shift). Still, many believe the fact that the penalty remains below the cost of insurance is why millions have chosen to simply pay the penalty and *just say no.*

Before the Affordable Care Act, 15 million Americans bought individual health insurance, which was typically more expensive and, unless you had a squeaky-clean health record, could be difficult to get. People who bought individual insurance often switched plans year to year and, because they had the bargaining power of only one person, had little leverage. Others chose to forgo health insurance altogether. The Affordable Care Act set out to change this, offering options to those buying individual health insurance and easing access to health insurance for the 40 million uninsured. Laws that adjust or replace the ACA will keep some of these goals, making individual insurance plans a real option, whereas before they were primarily a last resort.

Again, navigating the path that brings you the most *value* in healthcare requires recognizing when you have a choice and then making the best possible decision. In other words, you have to recognize when you are irrevocably drafted into a system and when you are a free agent. In the case of the ACA mandate, you are effectively drafted—as an American over age 18, you will pay a tax penalty if you fail to comply. However, the choice remains to "pull an Elway" and thumb your nose at the system that drafted you. Is refusing to be drafted the best choice? It depends on how much you're willing to pay for your ideology. But if you're looking at money and health, the answer is almost certainly no: in this situation (or until laws change), by admitting that you're drafted onto the team of Americans who use insurance to share the cost of medical bills, you get something for your money, as opposed to gifting $695 to the IRS.

A major way the ACA tries to offer choice to individuals, and that future laws will almost certainly continue to offer choice, is through the creation of "exchanges" or "marketplaces" where people who are not drafted can compare insurance plans to see if they qualify for subsidies to bring down the cost. And yet a central feature of the ACA was meant to be choice—at the federal and state-run marketplaces or exchanges, people would shop for health insurance like buying a plane ticket, as easy as using Kayak. The idea was that consumers would be able to buy plans optimized for their individual needs and that competition in these marketplaces would drive down the overall cost of insurance. The idea wasn't out of the blue. For years, individuals and small businesses have shopped for plans on private insurance exchanges—basically, the exchanges gave people and businesses without a lot of negotiating power the opportunity to sign onto bigger teams.

We've seen two ways the ACA tried to shepherd people into making the choice to get insurance—Medicaid expansion and tax penalty—and the third strategy was subsidizing health insurance through these exchanges. If you earn between 138 to 400 percent of the Federal Poverty Level, tax subsidies would offset the cost of health insurance (but only if you purchased new insurance on an exchange). The subsidy largely worked: 85 percent of the 5 million people who signed up for health insurance on the exchanges in the first year got some subsidy.

This chapter is a guide to these exchanges and market-places for you undrafted free agents who end up having the most choice of all. First, let's look at the different kinds of exchanges and then we'll explore how to shop at Healthcare. gov in more detail below.

## Marketplaces

After adoption of the Affordable Care Act, some states chose to set up their own marketplaces, also called "exchanges," and some states chose not to. This idea of shopping around for insurance in a more-free marketplace is likely to stick around, no matter what happens to the ACA. This means that if you are an unrestricted free agent, you may enroll for individual health insurance at your state's exchange (which can be found by searching online for "state exchanges") or if you discover that your state doesn't have an exchange of its own, you may enroll at the federal health insurance website, Healthcare.gov. Despite the disastrous rollout, Healthcare.gov has ironed out most of its technical glitches and is pretty easy to use. If you can book your own plane tickets at websites like Kayak.com, you should be able to navigate Healthcare.gov. According to ACA rules, if you or your family makes less than four times the federal poverty level, you are eligible for a subsidy, meaning that the government will pay a portion of your insurance costs. If you make below the federal poverty level, you are generally drafted onto the Medicaid team (or may in the future be offered a comparable lump-sum payment) and if you make more than four times the level, you will likely have to cover the cost of health insurance without a government subsidy.

## Private Exchanges

Even before the ACA, individuals could visit exchanges to purchase health insurance. These private exchanges were effectively the same as working with an insurance broker, allowing you to shop around, compare, and purchase insurance from a range of providers. Now in the post-ACA era, you are still able to use private exchanges but only by applying through ACA Marketplaces (Healthcare.gov) can you be eligible for federal subsidies. Also, as we've seen, instead of setting up employee health insurance plans, some companies are choosing to give employees money to spend toward the purchase of individual health insurance. This can get very complicated and is subject to complex rules. According to Obamacare Facts, businesses may be charged $100 a day for this arrangement, but companies like ZaneBenefits make a good alternative. Businesses should consult an expert and the IRS on this approach. With the adoption of the ACA, these private exchanges are usually only a good option for individuals buying insurance whose high income disqualifies them from federal subsidies and for whatever reason prefer working with a private exchange rather than with Healthcare.gov.

## Insurance Alternatives

In addition to the established mechanics of modern insurance, there are some unique insurance-like products that harken back to the days of community sharing. For example, Medi-Share is a Christian-based medical-expense-sharing ministry, and other community-, religious-, and membership-based options exist to spread risk across a population. That said, Medi-Share is not really "insurance" and I would suggest carefully exploring the networks, costs, and limitations of these alternative insurance strategies before depending on any one of these options for your health.

## How to Buy Health Insurance at Healthcare.gov

President Obama was right: when Healthcare.gov went live in 2013, it was a mess. Long waits and interrupted enrollments were just the start of the problems. "I mean, we fumbled the rollout on this healthcare law, when I do some Monday morning quarterbacking on myself," he said. "So again, these are two fumbles on something that—on a big game—but the game is not over."

But Obama was right about another thing: using the language of football, the government had fumbled but the game was not over. Now Healthcare.gov and the ACA market-place have made a huge recovery. With the exception of very rare glitches, the website is fast, well organized, and easy to use. Give it a try and it will lead you through the enrollment process. For those of you who want to look at film before game day, here are some tips for using Healthcare.gov.

### ENROLLMENT PERIOD

With a few exceptions, you can only buy individual health insurance plans during the open enrollment period, which is usually October 1 to January 31. One exception is for people with life-changing events, for example moving or changing jobs, or having a child, or getting a divorce. Another exception is for Medicaid enrollment. Both of these circumstances allow you to enroll in health insurance at any point during the year. (The SHOP small-business program also allows employers to enroll their employees at any time.) If you visit Healthcare.gov outside the open enrollment period, the system will prompt you to enter information to see if you qualify to sign up outside the enrollment window.

## WINDOW SHOPPING

You don't have to wait until you're ready to enroll before visiting Healthcare.gov. It's also a fine place to window shop, exploring the site to see what options might be available to you. A quick search for the terms "healthcare see plans" will take you to a link where you can compare plans at Healthcare.gov or will direct you to a similar resource on your state's exchange.

## ENTERING YOUR DATA

Most of the data required to apply for health insurance at Healthcare.gov is self-explanatory. When it's not, the site usually offers explanations. Here are some of the most common sticking points that you might want to discover or decide before you visit the site:

- ▶ Income is your household income, which includes your spouse's income.
- ▶ If you want, you can enter your doctors, your hospitals, and your medications. This will help to ensure that the care you want is included in the plan you buy, but before making a final decision, it's worth calling your doctor and/or specialists to double-check that they still accept the plan you are considering.
- ▶ To help the system suggest the best plan for your personal circumstances, enter your estimated healthcare costs (low, medium, high) with explanations of each.
- ▶ Consider seeing what plans come up before using the filters to refine your options. For example, after entering my basic information, Healthcare.gov returned 50 options. Then when I used filters like total cost, my doctors and medications, the list shrank to five.

## Choosing Your Plan Level

Just like an NFL player has some choice in how he is paid—a lower fixed amount with higher incentive pay, or a higher fixed amount with lower incentive pay—you have some choice in how you pay for your health insurance and healthcare. How and when you pay is determined largely by the "color" of the plan you choose—bronze, silver, gold, or platinum. Even with laws adjusting the ACA, the idea of levelled plans will continue. These levels are a stark example of the trade-off you will make when choosing any insurance: the higher the premium the less OOPs!, and the lower the premium the more the OOPs!. In this case, the lowest-level "bronze" plan has the lowest premium but will cost the most to use, whereas the highest-level "platinum" plan has the highest premium but you will pay less out-of-pocket to use it. The ACA limited yearly OOPs to $7,150 for individuals or $14,300 for families enrolled in bronze-level plans. Silver, gold, and platinum plans limited these OOPs! even further. There were also OOPs! limits for people whose earnings put them under certain income limits—as rules change, Healthcare.gov should still be able to lead you through the ins and outs of these specifics.

Another way to look at these plan levels is in terms of risk. The higher your premium, the lower your risk of being hit with a large healthcare bill. In that case, you pay more every month for the peace of mind that comes with the insurance company accepting the lion's share of the risk. On the other hand, a lower premium comes with higher personal risk—if you don't use your plan very much, you might be better off... but if Lady Luck takes a nasty turn, you will bear much of the responsibility for focused care. This isn't to mention high deductible plans, which are even below the ACA bronze level. If you are younger than 30 years old, the high deductible plan will fulfill the individual insurance mandate and help you avoid the penalty, but don't break a leg! If you're older than 30, forget it—federal rules are stacked against your use of a high-deductible plan.

Once you're in the ballpark (or stadium...) click "compare" on the plans you think are the frontrunners. Which plans cover chiropractic, glasses, mental health, or acupuncture? Do you prefer an HMO or a PPO? Are your doctors, hospitals, specialists, and medications covered? Now you can see all this information in an easy-to-read table, letting you compare apples to apples to make the best choice from among the remaining options.

## Pitfalls of the Marketplaces

My sister bought a plan on the ACA exchange only to find that her son's specialist was not on the plan. He needed critical medication and she had to scramble to find a new specialist who could prescribe the drug he needed. In other words, Healthcare.gov can make buying health insurance so easy that you can overlook some of the specifics. Don't let yourself click the "buy" button before you do your homework! Make sure your doctors and specialists and hospitals are in network on the plans you choose.

Another possible pitfall of the exchanges like the ACA Marketplace is that the shelves are getting a little thin. Major insurers like United Healthcare and Aetna are dropping out of the Marketplace due to losses. These exits leave the four states of Alabama, Alaska, South Carolina and Wyoming with only one insurer. What is a Marketplace without choice?

Premiums have continued to climb year after year for plans on the Marketplace, as well. Premium analysis from the Kaiser Family Foundation estimated an overall 9 percent increase in premiums for the second lowest "Silver" plans since the Marketplace was established. These rising premiums may be needed to offset insurer's losses for offering these plans. Basically, the ACA was built on the premise that young healthy patients would pay for insurance at a higher rate than they need to support the team of sicker patients paying less than their care actually costs. In this model, the individual mandate was supposed to ensure that cheap patients and expensive patients meet in the middle. Actually, they didn't meet in the exact middle—the overpayment of cheap patients would never offset the under-payment by expensive patients and so government stepped in to cover this gap, offering incentives to insurers to cover the costs of these very expensive patients. It's like NFL revenue sharing. Teams like Green Bay that play in a small media market get a boost from teams like New England that play in huge markets (remember Rich McKay citing this sharing as one secret of the NFL's success). However, Congress has blocked some of these government payments meant to help insurers cover the costs of putting expensive people on their plans. This leaves insurers high and dry and leads to insurers choosing to leave the system. You gotta love politics, right? Expect the debate over how and how much the government should subsidize healthcare to continue far into the future, no matter who is in the White House.

## Future of the Marketplace

The ACA Marketplace has been the political lightning rod for the law from its inception. At the core of this debate has been whether the federal government could mandate that individual citizens have health insurance and also subsidize the ability of lower income Americans to purchase this insurance. As you know, these fights have already made their way to the U.S. Supreme Court, and I wouldn't be surprised to see additional fights in the high court in years to come.

In addition to or perhaps as a result of legal struggles, pieces of the Marketplace haven't worked as intended. Basically, the ACA makes a big bet that young, healthy people who are forced by the mandate to pay into the system will help to cover the costs of older, more expensive people (with federal dollars helping to cover the costs of Medicaid, CHIP, and other low-income programs). Unfortunately, even with government programs designed to inject money into the Marketplace, the money that people pay into the system hasn't yet balanced the cost of healthcare going out. This balance scale tips against insurance companies—when bills exceed premiums and cost sharing, health insurers lose money. According to the *Wall Street Journal*, insurer United Healthcare lost almost $500 million on its 2016 ACA plans.

This means that costs and rates are likely to change, both on the side of your premiums and OOPs, and also on the side of how much insurers will ask from doctors and hospitals for specific treatments. With the exception of Missouri, Oklahoma, Texas, and Wyoming, the ACA gave states oversight for rate increases. States haven't had much luck keeping premiums level and now with Blue Cross/Blue Shield requesting a 60 percent increase in Texas in 2017, the federal government will get its chance to see if it can do what states couldn't and hold premiums at earlier levels.

Another strategy insurers are using to limit their costs is aggressively negotiating what they will pay for procedures and medicines. This leads to losing those previously in-network options that refuse to lower their prices, and leads to narrower networks and limited choices of doctors and hospitals for healthcare consumers. I worry that this will lead to patients leaving their known healthcare teams in favor of lower insurance premiums, leading to discontinuity in care.

And this doesn't even touch the glaring problem that despite the promise of universal healthcare, insurance remains unavailable to the very poor and—according to the Urban Institute—middle class families who buy coverage at Healthcare.gov spend nearly 25 percent of their income on premiums and OOPs!.

Most experts think that no matter if the White House and Congress are red or blue, some form of the programs initiated by the ACA are here to stay. The insurance mandate, subsidies, eligibility for Medicare and Medicaid, premiums, and plans may change, but the idea of government-managed health insurance with the goal of universal or near-universal coverage will continue into the future, no matter the name of the law under which they are implemented. Many of the specifics in this book will shift. But the fundamentals stay the same: Know when you are drafted and when you are a free agent; if you can, pick your healthcare team first and then figure out what insurance plans let you use these people and facilities; decide whether you prefer to pay more in premiums with less OOPs! or less in premiums with more OOPs!; and do your homework before making what seems like a little choice but can turn out to be a life-changing decision.

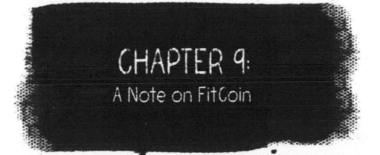

# CHAPTER 9:
## A Note on FitCoin

Some players refer to the NFL as "Not For Long," recognizing that due to injuries and competition from younger, faster players careers can be short. This means that in the NFL, health is wealth—the more a player can stay in front of, rather than behind injury, the longer he can stay healthy and the more wealth he can earn over his career. More and more insurance companies, employers, and health systems are recognizing the same thing; instead of paying a lot to fix the things that are wrong with a patient, they can pay much less to prevent those things from happening in the first place. Corporate wellness programs have been around for decades with mixed success. But now there's a new strategy to get you to eat well, stop smoking, and exercise. Now the federal government may be willing to pay you for it. You've heard of the Internet currency Bitcoin and I call the healthcare equivalent **FitCoin**—basically, the system that would have to pay for your healthcare may be willing to pay you for behaviors that make you less likely to use healthcare. The NFL has long had expert doctors and trainers tasked with keeping its employees fit, but other employers have, until now, been focused not on keeping employees fit but only on patching them back up once they're sick or injured.

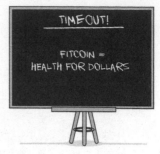

A Gallup poll found that eighty-six percent of American workers are overweight or have a chronic condition, leading to 450 million days of work lost costing up to $225 billion in lost productivity. The Affordable Care Act tried to change this, offering employees the ability to offset 30 percent of their healthcare premiums for weight loss or behavioral health programs or up to 50 percent off premiums if tobacco cessation is included. Depending on the cost of your plan and the state of these rules moving forward, this means that wellness could earn you thousands of dollars. As the political focus changes from the ACA to other systems, your incentive for wellness could come more from the idea of being able to keep any money you save on healthcare. Think about it: With an HSA, you put money into an account to use for a rainy day. If your lifestyle choices hold off this rainy day, that money in your HSA is yours. The gist is that no matter if the money comes as an incentive from the federal government or as the incentive to save money in your HSA, new models of healthcare will include ways to earn Fitcoin.

According to a survey by the Kaiser Family Foundation in partnership with the Health Research & Educational Trust, 89 percent of businesses with more than 200 employees offer some sort of incentivized wellness program. My own insurance offers $500 toward yearly premiums for meeting body mass index goals and pays money toward a monthly gym membership. To me this is like free money. Take advantage of these plans if your company has them—in this case, TEAM and "me" align as healthy employees save companies money in productivity and healthcare costs while the individual benefits from better health.

Medicare is testing these value-based, incentivized wellness programs in several states. In these programs, patients can win money or offset their premiums if they do certain things like get screening tests. Again, this is a win-win, with the system saving money by catching conditions when they are less expensive to treat and patients finding health problems before they get out of hand. Conversely, doctors and hospitals can lose money if patients don't get these screenings or act in other ways that promote health. On both the patient and doctor sides of these programs, there need to be ways to measure compliance. If Medicare is going to pay people to get a screening test, there has to be a way to document who actually gets these tests. And doctors are eventually going to want to say, "Hey, that was the patient's fault. I told her the right play but she didn't execute in the game!"

Eventually, healthcare and patients alike would like to measure the success of their wellness activities based on patient-centered goals. In other words, if healthcare helped you reach your own, very personalized goals, you could earn FitCoin. This will require even more involved health monitoring and data gathering, with your insurance company watching and evaluating very personal aspects of your life.

In this effort, healthcare could learn a thing or two from the NFL. Some teams have started putting computer chips in players' helmets to keep track of, for example, how far they move during practice plays. But some players have learned to game the system. Once when Saints coach Sean Payton asked his linemen why they were walking in circles during practice, they told him they just needed to get their numbers up!

Apparently, this level of monitoring is spanning the world. My wife's chiropractor plays professional rugby in the Philippines but only travels there for the season. During the rest of the year, the team gives him chips to wear in a wristband and in his shoes to monitor that he is running a certain number of sprints every day. He told me that he once got a call from his coach across the world asking why he didn't run the previous night!

With everyone from your employer to your insurer wanting you to be healthy, beware the ways in which you will be watched in the future. My health insurance company offers a health coach with my plan. Once I was eating pizza and drinking beer on a Saturday afternoon when my coach called and I was like, "How did you know I was being bad?!" This one was coincidence but that won't always be the case. In the future, your health insurance costs may be tied to chips monitoring everything from heartbeats to happy meals. Already some companies are incorporating Fitbits and Jawbones and other wearables into their wellness programs. According to an article in the *Wall Street Journal*, 40 to 50 percent of employers with wellness programs use various kinds of reporting to monitor their employees' progress. Unlike the NFL, these reporting devices most often are optional, but there is no law against mandating them—if you want the benefits and cash back offered by your wellness program, you might need to give up some of your privacy to get it.

If you make that bargain, make sure you understand the rules and what the data can be used for. Can your wellness program data be taken into account when evaluating you for raises and promotions? Find out if you are required to be tracked while out of the office or off duty. If your wellness program uncovers health issues, are you required to notify your company? These privacy concerns are huge questions that need to be answered in the coming years. Why? Because in these pay-for-performance models, the TEAM's bottom line will depend on knowing what the "me's" are doing and, more importantly, not doing with their health. In this way, your workplace is becoming like the NFL—when your fitness matters, self-reporting to your employer may not be enough.

In addition to the mechanics and privacy concerns of massive amounts of personal data being used to track your health is the question of what to do with this data. Imagine that a PCP (Primary Care Physician) practice has 5,000 patients who track blood pressure twice a day, blood sugar three times per day, and also chart the distance they walk or run each day. That's six data points per person, per day or 30,000 measurements that will hit this PCP's database every single day. This isn't even taking into account the endless possibilities for new data sources including heart rate monitors and new gadgets that track data from inside patients' bodies. Even now, there are many third-party companies that have ways to link your Fitbit with your PCP, but many PCPs don't want this data. What would they do with it? Like the transition from paper to electronic medical records, few PCP offices are equipped to handle the sea of data that can come from technologies that track wellness. With doctors stretched thin, learning a new software that visualizes patient data seems like just one more thing added to an already overly full schedule.

However, again like the transition to electronic medical records, wellness-tracking and wellness programs incentivized by various forms of FitCoin is the way of the future. It's not likely that you will ever generate *less* data than you do now. And as systems improve to help healthcare use this data, more insurers, employers, hospitals, and doctors will learn to take advantage of it. Right now, these programs are a little "Wild West" but in the future, they will be the norm. Remember, done right they can be a win–win with the TEAM aligning with the "me's." On the cutting edge of FitCoin, you can earn money for doing things that make you healthier. What's better than that?

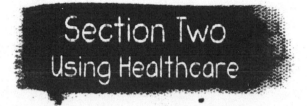

# Section Two
## Using Healthcare

Congratulations and welcome to your healthcare team! Whether you were drafted into your insurance or chose it as a free agent, you now have some financial security for your healthcare costs. Unfortunately, choosing insurance was only the start. Like the NFL, getting on the team is only the beginning. Now it's time to play the game.

There are many places or settings in which the game of healthcare is played, each with their own unique elements. Once upon a time, if you wanted to watch football you had to go to the stadium. Now you can watch at home or on one of a dozen handheld devices, usually interacting with other fans via one of these second or third screens. The healthcare experience has evolved as well. Now you can get care not only in your PCP's office or hospital, but also in urgent cares, free-standing ERs, surgery centers, skilled nursing facilities, virtual offices, and more. Healthcare is trying to push everyone to the least intensive and expensive level for better value, both in quality and cost, and this means the ongoing addition of options. For example, New Mexico is even trying to bring the entire hospital team to patients at home. Procedures that used to take three days in a hospital are being done in surgery centers and you are home that evening. Like choosing how you want to experience the NFL, each of these healthcare settings has pros and cons, making it a very personal choice.

These settings are also being increasingly monitored, rated, and evaluated. Doctors and hospitals in these models send surveys to you and their scores matter. I was fortunate enough to get a tour of Levi's Stadium, the new home of the San Francisco 49ers, before it opened. Former player and now Vice-President of Communications Bob Lange explained the data they collected before, as he put it, "opening the flood gates of experience" for fans. Like healthcare wants to build better hospitals and surgery centers, the 49ers wanted to build a smarter stadium, full of apps and wireless access and ways to navigate to your seat and make sure your food shows up when you want it. The stadium would include a museum and a five-star restaurant, not to mention solar panels and judicious water usage.

This same enhanced experience movement has hit healthcare. This section will break down the many settings where the actual game of healthcare is played. With choice comes challenge—now with a spectrum of options for where to receive care, you have to pick the one that's best for your needs. This section explores how.

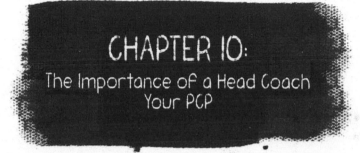

# CHAPTER 10:
## The Importance of a Head Coach
### Your PCP

"I am tired all the time, something just isn't right," my father told me on the phone one day. He shared that on his lunch break he had started taking naps in his truck to get through the day. This was not my dad. As one who never missed a day of work or even took a lunch break, sleeping at work would be the height of laziness.

I first thought his fatigue must be a side effect of one of his medications or the result of a combination that wasn't working. I had a professor in med school who taught me the quirky acronym FTD-TPUP, which stood for "First Think Drugs, Then Pick Up the Phone." It meant that when a patient experienced a symptom, they should first consider the chance it was a side effect of one of their medications, and then if it can't be explained away as a necessary evil, call their primary care physician (PCP). On the phone with my dad, we started the

"FTD" part. He stumbled through his medications by memory, and none seemed like the culprit. I knew he was seeing many specialists: an endocrinologist for his diabetes, a cardiologist for his low blood pressure while standing, a gastroenterologist and oncologist for esophageal cancer that was in remission, a urologist for kidney stones, and his ophthalmologist for diabetic eye disease. But I asked him the million-dollar question: Who is your PCP? Of course, like many of the patients I see in the hospital, he did not have one.

When I was growing up, we would play football in the backyard and we had a play called "everybody go long." It was a chaotic cacophony of kids running as far and as fast as they could while screaming for the ball. This was my dad's healthcare. His cancer doctors are at Emory, part of a completely different healthcare system than his endocrinologist. His urologist is a private provider, not part of any larger system, and his gastroenterologist is part of his smaller local hospital. They all have different electronic medical records or computerized medical record systems—all except for the urologist who still uses good old paper charts. He was caught between the fragmented and uncoordinated team of teams.

When Dad needs an MRI, he has to go to one of three different locations, depending on which of his specialists ordered it. CAT scans and blood work follow the same illogical process. Once he traveled all the way to Florida to have his cataracts fixed only to find that the surgeon's office didn't have the clearance letter from his endocrinologist.

My dad needed a head coach—a home base for all his information and a person who could synchronize his care while looking at the big picture. Ignoring my advice, he instead made the rounds to all of his specialists including his cancer doctor who all said that his fatigue was not due to their disease. He was relieved to hear the cancer was at bay. Then his endocrinologist finally did the work of a PCP. He asked to go over all his medications one more time. Looking at all the different specialists and lists of medications it became clear that his gastroenterologist had started him on a drug called Reglan for persistent heartburn, a fact he had forgotten when we had reviewed his meds over the phone. He was to take it only as needed, up to three times per day, but given my dad's obsessive nature he took it religiously, needed or not. That was the culprit. In addition to making him drowsy, overuse of the drug had affected his brain and nervous system. He stopped the drug but unfortunately some of his symptoms have not gone away.

Could we have nipped his use of this drug in the bud if he had had a PCP? My guess is yes.

Unfortunately, my dad is not the only one who eschews a PCP in favor of a team of disconnected specialists. Fifty percent of men aged 18 to 50 don't have a PCP and a third haven't had a checkup in a year according to an *Esquire* survey. It is not just men—my aunt who is in her fifties just admitted she recently got a PCP for the first time, after going to give blood and finding that the top number of her blood pressure was 180. Her new PCP started her on medication but the scary part is that she has probably had high blood pressure for years. Her new PCP also recommended that she see a dermatologist to have a mole evaluated. The mole turned out to be melanoma, but because her PCP helped her catch it early, it was still very treatable.

My mother on the other hand has had the same PCP since 1998 despite his not having privileges at her hospital of choice (a tradeoff we talked about in selecting your healthcare team). She correctly placed her PCP over choice of hospital because she rarely is in the hospital. Also, she knows the hospitalist who will step in for her PCP in the hospital and knows that both her PCP and the hospitalist are committed to make a smooth handoff. In a recent visit my mom's PCP noticed she was wearing reading glasses and asked, "Who is your eye doctor?" He wanted to make sure this new team member was in the know about my mom's health concerns and also felt able to share new information with the PCP. All her specialists send their records to her PCP's office, which office staff ensures happens before my mom's visits. As a social worker herself, Mom knows the results of communication gaps. Her PCP ensures these gaps don't occur in her healthcare.

This kind of care coordination can be as or more important than the care itself. Without a head coach for your healthcare team there will be a lot of "everybody-going-long" on your team. You probably have felt like you are the one going long—long hours of trying to coordinate all this yourself! A recent *Vox* article showed that being a patient can easily be the equivalent of a full-time job. A good PCP, like a good coach, can protect you and hopefully save you some time and energy.

Having a PCP is more than a luxury. There is medical evidence that good primary care improves health and lowers cost. The Affordable Care Act recognized the importance of PCPs, conceptualizing the teams of new healthcare with the head coach of a PCP at their center. For example, the ACA creates Patient Centered Medical Homes (PCMH), a model in which the PCP is paid extra to coordinate care and if they are able to save money in addition to meeting quality measures, the PCP keeps some of the savings. PCP offices have to earn a certification to become a PCMH, which includes meeting six criteria including practicing team-based care and being patient-centered in addition to coordinating care. There is evidence that this model improves quality but less data on reducing cost. You can ask your PCP office if they are a PCMH.

Another model reinforced by the Affordable Care Act that centers on PCPs is Accountable Care Organizations (ACOs). In an ACO, a team of doctors and hospitals and other health organizations come together to share data and practices to improve the value of care. If your PCP is in an ACO then you are automatically drafted into the model. While ACOs are limited to organizations that provide care to more than 5,000 patients and are thus most common in systems that manage Medicare patients, Medicare Advantage and even private insurers have started ACOs as well. Like the PCMH model in which a PCP can earn a portion of monies saved, the members of an ACO are allowed to divvy up 50 percent of the organization's savings over a certain benchmark. Patrick Conway, M.D., Chief Medical Officer for the Centers for Medicare and Medicaid services, shared with me that ACOs are specifically meant to foster teamwork between the healthcare team and patients seeking better outcomes at a lower cost. In fact, he felt PCMHs were designed to encourage the patient to be part of the healthcare decision-making process.

Now, do you remember our most important measure of successful healthcare: value. In the value equation, value is quality divided by cost. We've seen how PCPs are central to healthcare's attempts to save cost. But where is the quality? Didn't we learn our lesson about cutting costs at the expense of quality from the managed care debacle of the 1990s? Luckily, quality is written into the new rules, too. To earn payouts from a PCHM or ACO, in addition to saving money, a doctor has to meet 32 quality standards many of which deal with patient outcomes. So here's another way your PCP is like your coach: he or she has income tied to the results of the game.

I asked Dr. Conway about where patients fit into these models. Basically, he said that the goal of Medicare and other government-run programs is to align doctors' incentives with patients' goals. He shared that actual, patient-centered goals, like being able to see a child's soccer game, would be the best markers to set as healthcare goals but that we are not there yet in terms of measuring these kinds of things in a standard manner. For now, he is focused on the idea that when the overall quality of your care increases and your overall own cost goes down, then the TEAM and the "me" align and, like an NFL team, everyone wins.

Like the bar in Cheers, your PCP office is a place where, "everybody knows your name." According to the CDC, this is where most healthcare happens, with 928.6 million PCP office visits a year. New programs and new regulations are starting to put in writing what the world of healthcare has known for years: When you have a PCP, everyone wins. Healthcare starts here. If you don't have a PCP, flip back to the chapter on choosing a doctor and then get to it. With a PCP managing your care, there's a better chance you'll have time to come back to read the rest of this book later.

# CHAPTER 11:
## Your Decision-Making Style
## Who Calls the Plays?

Hall of Fame 49ers head coach Bill Walsh told the *New York Times* about his early days as an assistant with the Cincinnati Bengals: "I used to fight tooth and nail right there on the sidelines with running backs coach Bill Johnson. He wanted to call all runs. If it was left up to me, we'd be dropping back there and throwing downfield all of the time." He goes on to say that Bill Johnson was the running backs coach—Johnson was trying to prove his philosophy that running the ball was the best way to win games. Walsh had a passing background and was trying to prove his philosophy that throwing the ball was the way to put points on the board.

"If you get a coach calling the plays who's trying to prove his philosophies in his area, you're in trouble," Walsh said.

I see this all the time in healthcare—the surgeon wants to do surgery, the physical therapist wants to do physical therapy, and any number of specialists want to reach for whatever promising, new drug is on the top of the shelf. Each wants what he or she thinks is best for the patient, only their judgment is clouded by their frame of reference. As a doctor, you absolutely have to believe that you can make a difference. Otherwise, you just can't get up in the morning and do your job. But coming to think you're the only one who can make a difference or that you have the best answer for every patient in every situation is one source of bad play-calling in healthcare. You can't run the ball all the time. You can't throw the ball all the time. It's the ability to step back from ego-driven decision-making that's ultimately best for NFL teams and for patients.

That said, just like in football, no one decision-making method is best in every situation. In the NFL, sometimes the head coach or offensive coordinator listens to the input of all the virtual coaches in the team box who are running the numbers. Sometimes the coach goes with his gut, calling the play directly into the quarterback's helmet. And sometimes the coach or offensive coordinator gives the quarterback a set of options and lets the quarterback decide which play to run based on the way the defense lines up.

In his book, *Being Mortal*, the esteemed doctor and author Atwul Gwande describes three ways doctors and patients make decisions: patriarchal (the doctor makes decisions), informative (the doctor offers information but depends on the patient to make decisions), and a model in which patient and doctor collaborate on health decisions. Let's take a look at these three styles now.

## Patriarchal Decisions

Some patients want to be at the center of every medical decision. But some patients do not. It's worth asking yourself if you really want the responsibility of choice or if you would rather let the experts make choices for you. Asserting your agency in making medical decisions is a decision in itself. If you feel more comfortable deferring to your doctor or health-care team, there is nothing wrong with that. You may not feel that way about every decision but don't feel bad about letting your coaches have the final say on a call. Sometimes patients ask their doctors, "What would you do if you were me or if it were your mom?" This is another way of saying, "I trust you to make the call." If a doctor does not feel comfortable with this approach he or she should tell you. If it's an important decision that depends on personal preference, your doctor should push back against your impulse to outsource the choice. But be aware that it's perfectly reasonable, even in the current climate of patient empowerment and shared decision-making, to choose not to choose. You don't have to make every choice yourself. If it feels best to you, you can still defer to your doctors' opinions.

## Informative Style

When Tom Flores was the quarterback of the Raiders from 1960–1966, he called his own plays. When he coached the Raiders from 1979–1987, he asked his quarterbacks to take responsibility for play-calling as well. In Flores' model, coaches helped provide information, but it was up to the team's MVP and star quarterback to make the important choices. There's a similar decision-making model in healthcare, the "informative style," or what Dr. Gwande calls a "retail relationship." In this style, the doctor provides the expert information and then the patient decides what to do about it. Just as there is nothing wrong with patients deferring to their doctor, there is nothing wrong with doctors deferring to their patients, as long as the information the doctor provides includes his or her opinion of the most medically responsible decisions.

Jennifer Fong Ha notes in the *Ochsner Journal* that in the 1950s to 1970s, doctors used to keep information from their patients—for instance, it used to be common not to tell a patient he or she had cancer. This was to protect them from the bad news of an incurable disease. Now doctors are upfront with their patients. The emphasis is on patient empowerment and a patient's ability to get the care he or she thinks they need. Some healthcare thought leaders feel that giving patients all the choice of insurance plans and doctors and hospitals and tests and procedures, and even giving them more of the bill, will lead to more value. They may be right. But for this model of patient-as-an-informed-consumer-with-the-power-of-choice to work, patients need all the relevant information and the skills to evaluate it. I call this "comparency" or transparency with the ability to compare. With these two things, I am all for patients being the ultimate agents of healthcare choice.

Actually, even if you prefer doctors to shape your choices, you're going to have to dip into this informative style pretty often. Unless you're married to a doctor, you don't have the luxury (my wife would say the duty...) to bounce every question and decision off an expert. Most of your lifestyle choices are yours and yours alone.

But "informative style" decision-making can go too far, as well. A study showed that when people are confronted with a medical condition they believe might require care, 35 percent of patients try to self-diagnose on the internet before seeing their doctor. I'm all for self-sufficiency...but have you seen the state of medical information on the internet lately? I'm amazed anyone with a smartphone can leave their house for fear of succumbing to some horrible condition. Amazon might have gone a step too far when it sold mugs with the slogan, "Please don't confuse your Google search with my medical degree," but the point remains: there's a reason that doctors spend so many years in school. Making healthcare decisions is hard! Even if you keep control of the ultimate decisions affecting your health, it can be very useful to include a doctor's recommendations in the decision-making process.

## Shared Decision-Making

Writing about his father's doctor's use of shared decision-making, Atwul Gwande says, "Benzel [the doctor] saw himself as neither the commander nor a mere technician in this battle but instead as a kind of counselor and contractor on my father's behalf. It was exactly what my father needed."

This is shared decision-making, a mixture of patriarchal and informative styles in which the doctor gets the patient's preferences and then makes a strong suggestion for the treatment that would best align with his or her wishes. Decision-making in healthcare has been studied many ways, many times but one study I find especially compelling is one by the Agency for Healthcare Research and Quality that found that not only did shared decision-making result in a more positive patient experience, but that it actually increased the value of healthcare—when patients and doctors worked together to make decisions, costs came down and quality went up. Interestingly, one reason for this is that patients are sometimes able to decide against having tests and procedures that a doctor would order just to cover all the bases. A doctor who makes all the choices assumes all the risk. When a patient helps to make choices, the patient can accept some of the consequences for their actions and decide not to have that just-in-case MRI or that let's-rule-out-even-the-remote-possibility-of test.

It is in this model of shared decision-making that I see the doctor most like a coach. Good coaches can use many different approaches and can switch their play calling like a chameleon to match the needs of the individual players. They will push at certain points and step back at others. Similarly, players can adjust and push their coach. This is another reason why having a good PCP or head coach is so important. If your coach knows you and knows how you usually make decisions, he or she will know, for example, that when you insist on your decision, it's not just your informative style but also an instance in which you feel especially strong. When a coach knows a player's strengths and weaknesses the play is more likely to work.

This is how it works most of the time: Your preference influences how you and your doctor make a decision, but the situation influences how the decision is made, too. What it comes down to is the fact that no matter your preference, depending on your situation, you should be prepared to make decisions in any of the preceding styles. It is okay to defer to the coaches at times and to make the call yourself in others.

Communicate with your team and your healthcare team what your wishes and preferences are and be ready to make adjustments when your plays don't work.

Find what works for you. In the end, coach and patient should decide on a path forward, with both understanding the risks and benefits of the play-call.

And then there are situations that blow your usual decision-making process out of the water....

## Special Situations in Healthcare Decision-Making

### HOW MUCH TIME IS ON THE CLOCK?

There's one way decisions are made during the game and another way they're made with 28 seconds on the clock. In healthcare as in football, you might have an entire off-season to decide who will start at quarterback or less than 30 seconds to call the most important play of your career. When time is tight—at the end of a football game or in a health emergency—collaborative decision-making and the multidisciplinary input of a team of specialists can go out the window. In these cases, expect your coach to take over. With that in mind, it's critically important to get on the same page with your coach (your doctor) before there's an emergency. Your coach should know your goals. Your coach should know your physical, philosophical, spiritual, and psychological constraints. Then, when the clock is running out, your coach will have a better chance of calling the plays you want.

### DATA-DRIVEN DECISIONS

In the NFL, decisions are driven by data. Should a team kick a field goal or go for it on fourth down? You can bet that every NFL coach has a team of data nerds analyzing the numbers. How should a team use their all-important draft choices? The data that comes from players in the NFL Combine drives these decisions—what's a player's time in the 40-yard dash? How much can he bench and squat? What's his vertical jump? And if it takes five MRIs to get a clear understanding of an old knee injury, then you better believe that player's going to get five

MRIs. The NFL will go to any length to get the data it needs to win games.

Healthcare is also informed by data, both your personal data and by the data generated by other patients and by more basic scientific studies. Based on your health history, your genetic history, your current health, and your diagnosis, doctors can put together a pretty clear picture of what they think should happen next and what the outcomes are likely to be. But just like the process of decision-making as a whole is in a time of great transition, so too is medical data. Just because your information will supposedly be stored in a medical record system doesn't mean that it will be. When data is part of the decision-making process, keep your data with you—insist on keeping copies of all relevant information. Then wherever you are going, call ahead to make sure any new doctor or specialist or facility has the information it needs. Should you have to do this? No. But electronic medical records are not ready for prime time—data can and often is misplaced or lost entirely. At best, this can result in delay. At worst, the inadequacy of medical records can lead to dangerously bad decisions.

Finally, into this tangle of data you bring your preferences and wishes. Despite the data, your goals can point your health-care team's decisions in a completely different direction. Like a good NFL coach, your doctor may challenge or push you on your choices, usually aided by data. But at the end of the day, data has to take a backseat to your goals as a person.

## DECISIONS IN THE WAR ROOM

Former Baltimore Ravens head coach Brian Billick paints the picture of a "war room" on NFL draft day: doctors and owners and executives and general managers and scouts all bring their playbooks and opinions and strategies and goals. On draft day, the team makes *major* decisions. Expect a similar war room if you are ever confronted with a major healthcare decision. When a big choice has to be made, know when the war room will take place and prepare. You will want all your representatives there and don't forget to bring your own data. Ideally, the war room would be one critical meeting but given logistics, it may be stop-and-start, more-information-needed. It may require that the team discuss before revisiting the decision.

## One Obvious Choice

A couple years ago at a routine checkup with my PCP, we found that my blood pressure was at the very high end of normal. He correctly pointed out a recent study showing a stark difference in health outcomes between patients with low-normal and high-normal blood pressures. I needed to get my blood pressure down and the study implied that I needed to get it down fast. The obvious choice was blood pressure medication. It was a no-brainer.

Or was it? I asked a key question: Who were the people in this study? It turned out that many of the patients on this study had other risk factors for heart disease. I had none of these risk factors. While it was very dangerous for people on this study to have high blood pressure, it was less dangerous for me. This meant that instead of reaching right for medications, it was appropriate for me to try to manage my high blood pressure with lifestyle changes—losing weight, exercising, and managing my diet. I did and it's largely worked, reducing my blood pressure into the middle of the normal range.

Sometimes there are medical situations that have only one option. If you have meningitis, you should take antibiotics.

If you are bitten by a bat, you should have anti-rabies treatment. If you're bleeding, your healthcare team should stop the bleeding, for gosh sake. But, surprisingly, it turns out there are fewer of these no-brainer calls in healthcare than you would imagine. If a doctor states that medical evidence clearly leads to only one conclusion, ask if the patients that led to this evidence are just like you. Do they have the same values and preferences? Do they have the same goals? I'm not telling you to be difficult in the face of overwhelming evidence pointing to one obvious treatment. But even when a medical decision seems like a no-brainer, it's worth using your brain. Asking everyone involved in a medical decision to open their minds can at least help your team take a look at other possibilities.

## How to Make a Decision When There Is No Clear Option

According to the NFL news site *The Redzone*, in 1970 when he was offensive coordinator at UCLA, Dick Vermeil made a chart showing when to go for a two-point conversion after a touchdown. It had two columns: "lead by" and "trail by." Then for each point value, it told Vermeil to go for one or two. It was a simple chart that seemed like it should offer simple decisions. The reality is much more complicated. In her 2010 article, "Coaches Still Vexed by Going for Two," reporter Judy Battista tells of a decision by Colts coach Jim Caldwell, trailing by five points just before the half, who went for one even when the Vermeil chart said it was a clear time for two.

"The decision is so fraught with uncertainty, the gray area between right and wrong is so fuzzy, that even a Rutgers statistics professor who has analyzed 2-point play…wavered about what he would have done," Battista writes. In other words, even in the decisive arena of football, things are sometimes not as clear-cut as they seem.

Here's my experience of uncertainty in healthcare: On Tuesdays, I play trivia with a team and I'm terrified that eventually I will miss a medical question. Thankfully it hasn't happened yet. Doctors never want to be wrong. But in my opinion, it's time for doctors to embrace and discuss uncertainty. I cannot tell you how many times in my career my team has flip-flopped over what is the "scientifically best" option for a patient. The whole field of medicine does it too. Women should take hormones, no, they shouldn't; no we're wrong, they should take hormones after all; no, we we're wrong about being wrong...and on and on.

When there is no clear answer, the patient should hear the case for both sides and then turn to their preference—even if that preference is asking the doctor to decide. In fact, in the article by Yale doctor, Terri Fried, M.D., in the *New England Journal of Medicine*, she argues that when the evidence is not clear and there is uncertainty, that is precisely when doctors should offer the most direction. She goes on to say that doctors should share their thought process out loud, including patients in not only the information and the decision, but the process that leads from one to the other.

## WHEN THERE IS NO GOOD OPTION

There's another situation in which there is no clear best choice, and that's when there doesn't seem to be any good choice at all. For example, in the early days of the AIDS epidemic our only treatment was morphine for comfort. I will never forget my first day on the AIDS wards walking into my patients' rooms with little to offer as they suffered their death sentence, gaunt, emaciated, and without hope. In my opinion, these situations are no time to stop making decisions—in fact, I think it's the right time for doctors and patients to be more free with their decisions than ever before. If the patient or the doctor suggests less scientifically proven treatments, now is the time for the other person to agree. When it seems like no good options are on the table, it's time for a special kind of shared decision-making, one in which the doctor or the patient comes up with ideas and then the team decides to push forward together.

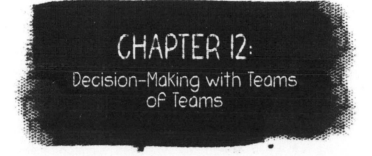

# CHAPTER 12:
## Decision-Making with Teams of Teams

In the previous chapter, you probably got the gist that the field of healthcare holds shared decision-making in high regard! But now the process of making healthcare decisions is shifting even further, from collaboration between patient and doctor to the interactive decisions of an entire healthcare team, ideally with the patient at its center. Instead of a one-on-one interaction, healthcare decisions are taking place in the fragmented chaos of "teams of teams." In this model, your doctor is like the head coach. The reality is that in this new model, you will have less time with your head coach, but this short time you have may be influenced by your interactions with the many others on the coaching staff—the offensive and defensive coordinators, a line coach, a receivers coach, and all the rest of the specialists that make up your healthcare team. Of course (and again!), when you add your insurer and the hospital and your agents and all the other players in this teams-of-teams system, it can be like NHL, NBA, and NFL teams all trying to coordinate on a concessions menu.

This Sunday's game may only be 11 actual minutes of football, but it's the result of a relentless schedule of meetings and practices and trainings. Some of those meetings are with the head coach, but most are not. In the first chapter of this book, we talked about the cooperation and sometimes competition between TEAM and me, but in this new model of shared decision-making in healthcare, it's really TEAM and we. Remember, this is new territory for doctors too! We doctors haven't had time to settle into the mechanics of this TEAM–we decision-making. There's almost never a sit-down with all of these teams in which a pathologist talks to the radiologist who talks with the endocrinologist and the cardiologist and the surgeon and the primary care physician. Instead, right now, it's an unusual system with a cadence of a critical few moments and logistical gaps separated by long delays.

Actually, there is exactly one disease with a history of sit-downs where doctors and specialists discuss their patients. Can you guess what it is? It's cancer. For years, cancer docs have gotten together in what are called "tumor boards" to coordinate their patients' care. The surgeon, oncologist, radiologist, and the lung doctor (in the case of lung cancer) all give their input, then one person carries the message back to the patient and a final decision on the direction of care is made. This model is migrating to other areas beyond cancer care. This is called a multidisciplinary approach and is much like the collaboration of the many different coaches, coordinators, doctors, trainers, and scouts of an NFL team.

Outside of cancer with its established history of tumor boards, it's not always practical to get all of a patient's doctors and specialists into the same room at the same time. Instead, hospitals use "huddles." The first football huddle happened in 1890 at Gallaudet University, a traditionally deaf university in Washington D.C., when the quarterback, Paul Hubbard, asked the offense to form a tight circle around him so the defense wouldn't see him signing the plays. I travel across the country helping to fix hospitals and hospitalist practices and I see that huddles are all the rage. There is a safety huddle, a case management huddle, a nursing huddle...there are huddles to plan new huddles. Used well, these huddles can be an important way for people on the healthcare side to coordinate their patients' care. Used poorly, these informal huddles are a stopgap that imperfectly replace real meetings. There's another danger to huddles, namely the possibility to cut you, the patient, out of the decision-making process.

Unfortunately, while the shift toward multidisciplinary teams results in all of your doctors getting together to talk about you, it can come at the expense of your own decision-making power. A recent study by Pola Hahlweg explained that, "The processes in multidisciplinary team meetings we observed did not exhibit shared decision-making. Patient perspectives were absent. If multidisciplinary team meetings wish to become more patient-centered they will have to modify their processes and find a way to include patient preferences in the decision-making process."

In other words, healthcare settled on its favorite kind of decision-making, one in which decisions are a collaboration between doctor and patient. And then the desire to include input from the multidisciplinary team blew this shared decision-making out of the water. Now we're in flux. Doctors don't quite know how to make decisions in the context of these new teams of teams. Patients don't know whether to sit back and have their doctors tell them what to do, or lean in and tell their *doctors* what to do. Because the field of healthcare is stuck in this middle ground between shared decision-making and multidisciplinary decisions without the patient's input, it can be your job (unfortunately) to make sure your voice is heard. Yes, the teams of teams that have a giant folder of data probably know what's best for most people. But you might not be "most people."

If your healthcare goal is to return to running competitive 10K races, maybe a cortisol shot in your arthritic knee isn't enough. Or if your goal is to die with dignity, maybe the most aggressive treatment against a terminal cancer isn't most appropriate. Your goals influence the "best" treatment but unless you add your voice to the decision-making conversation, your goals can be sidelined by a coach or coaches that want to do what's right but don't always know what that is.

How to coordinate and collaborate among these teams of doctors with you, the MVP of the healthcare team, at the center, is a major challenge facing the teams of teams in healthcare of the future. For now, you may have to be your own decision-making advocate. With each of these teams, being your own advocate looks a little different and takes place in a slightly different context. Following are general characteristics of decision-making within many of the teams you will work with in healthcare.

## Owner

Jerry Jones, owner of the Dallas Cowboys, has the final decision on whether or not to pay for a new quarterback. Like it or not sometimes your insurance company is your "owner" and makes the ultimate decision about what procedures and medications you can have. Of all the things that frustrate me about healthcare, this one is right up at the top of the list. In football, a coach can know darn well that his team needs a new offensive lineman to protect his quarterback's blind side. How frustrating is it when the owner says no, or commits the team to losing the first 8 games of the season before agreeing to buy the player the coach knew was needed all along? In healthcare, the owner doesn't always listen to the coach (the insurance company doesn't always do what the doctor says). You can be the most empowered patient in the world, but sometimes you can feel powerless against the decisions made by your owner. In the final section of this book, we'll talk about exactly what you can do to fight the decisions made by your insurance system. However, sometimes this is a losing cause. When the insurance company makes a decision, you, your coach, and the rest of the team either fight or make the most of it.

## PCP vs. Specialist

Just as some patients defer to their doctors to make the call on healthcare decisions, sometimes your PCP defers to specialists. This is like a head coach that is more offensive- than defensive-minded deferring to the judgment of the defensive coordinator. In healthcare and football, good coaches understand their limitations and will delegate decisions to people with more expertise and knowledge. But what this means is that instead of the decision happening between you and your coach, the decision can be "once-removed"—it can happen between doctor and specialist, with the doctor in charge of communicating a decision that has already been made.

Conversely, PCPs know a little about a lot—they know the basics of many conditions and so know enough to know when to ask specialists to join the team. There are a couple dangers in this relationship between PCP and specialist and one of them is the possibility for your PCP to try to handle something beyond their scope. There can even be incentives in new managed care systems for PCPs to keep the specialists out. A common saying in safety is "don't blame the individual, blame the system." But while sitting in the doctor's office, you're not going to change the system of managed care incentives and so the best thing you can do is keep a close eye on the individual. Keep your antenna out for a head coach making decisions that require the expertise of a line coach. If you think your PCP is making calls that require a specialist, ask for a second opinion.

## Nurse Practitioners and Physician Assistants

In the NFL, trainers are in the trenches delivering most of the care, under the supervision of the team doctor. As healthcare moves to this team model, you will be seeing more and more of the equivalent of these valuable team members, your nurse practitioner or physician's assistant. In fact, 19 states now allow nurse practitioners to practice independently, acting as head coaches. Just like a PCP, if a nurse practitioner knows when to bring specialists onto the team, this can be a very successful arrangement. Also, some independent nurse practitioners consult with a doctor, adding a layer of oversight. There are great and excellent doctors and some not so good ones. It is the same for NPs and PAs. And just like working with your PCP, if you feel uncomfortable with your NP's or PA's experience level, be upfront and ask to include someone with more expertise in your decisions.

## Hospital or Facility

If you receive treatment in a hospital or nursing home or other healthcare facility, the facility will be involved in your decisions. Hospitals have many layers of professionals including case managers, physical therapists, and pharmacists, not to mention nurses and medical assistants, and sometimes medical students or trainees. At the top there are Chief Medical Officers and an entire suite of executives including CEOs, CFOs, COOs, and on and on. Think of all these members of the hospital team as the business or front office of an NFL team.

The front office's job is to make sure the system of the team runs smoothly, and this includes making sure the team is in the black. This means that a facility needs to take in as much money as it pays out. A hospital might get some money from you, but chances are the bulk of its payments come from insurance companies. This can influence how the facility makes decisions. For instance, if your insurance will only pay for a two-night stay, the hospital has a strong incentive to get you out the door after two nights. Again, conflicts in decision-making between a hospital and an insurance company can be similar to the conflicts between your doctor and an insurance company—it can be the conflict between what's best for you and what "good enough" treatment an insurance plan can offer for much less cost.

Hospitals also decide what treatments they offer and which medications are on the formulary—the weapons we doctors have to fight your diseases. The availability of treatments and the need for hospitals to work within the constraints of patients' insurance companies can put doctors at odds with their own hospital. As you can guess, this makes a confusing and often frustrating decision-making atmosphere. You want treatment that meets your goals. Your doctor wants treatment that aligns with specialists' opinions, meets your goals, and is also possible in the system of insurance and hospital. Your insurance wants to treat you effectively and inexpensively. And your hospital wants to treat you within the boundaries allowed by insurance. Of course, if you pull back this first curtain of incentives, you can find a million more. In some cases, all of these incentives align, these teams work together, and the decisions that are made really do help you along the path to your healthcare goals. Other times, mismatched incentives combine with people in this system who prioritize incentives over your healthcare goals, and the path takes unfortunate twists and turns.

## Your Family or Other "Agents"

In the middle of my wife's surgery for a twisted bowel, her surgeon came out to the waiting area where I was sitting with family. She was still under anesthesia and the surgeon was carrying a few photos. "See her gallbladder? Look at that scarring," he pointed out. I have seen many gallbladders and could see that my wife's needed to come out. After a quick discussion, the surgeon and I agreed it was the right thing to do and he went back into the theater to perform the operation. Ideally, this would have been discussed with my wife but in this case of an unforeseen issue with her under anesthesia and thus not able to be part of the decision-making process, it was up to her agent, me, to make the call.

Similarly, my siblings and I have conference calls to discuss my dad's health and healthcare decisions. Usually, I talk directly to his team of doctors and report back to him and then also report to my sisters so that we can make sure both of my dad's teams work together.

Let's hope that your family members are able to help you make healthcare decisions with your goals and only your goals in mind. Especially if you are incapacitated, your spouse or siblings or children or other people who are close to you may have to make important choices. Like a sports agent, they may have to negotiate for you, coming to a "deal" with all the people on the healthcare side. If you have one agent, decision-making is pretty straightforward. But many of us have multiple people looking out for us. That's great! The more love and concern, the better. But it can also lead to confused decision-making. Will your spouse or your sister have the final say in your healthcare decisions? Do you expect your team of agents to collaborate on a decision or do you want one person to make the call?

To avoid fuzzy decision-making right when you need it least, work to define how your team of agents will help you make or independently make your healthcare decisions. This can mean designating one person with durable power of attorney or defining your medical surrogate. Realize that if you don't designate who will make decisions, the default is your next of kin. As a doctor, I cannot tell you how many times we contact a long lost relative who is forced to make an important medical decision for someone they barely know, when standing right beside that patient's bedside is a friend or partner with much more experience. The gist is, if you're going to be in the hospital (and even if you're not!), make sure you define the person or persons who will make decisions for you. And then make sure these people know their roles and how you expect them to work together to ensure you get the care you truly want.

# CHAPTER 13:
## Game P.L.A.N.S. – How to Execute Your Game-Day Strategy

Former Philadelphia Eagles and now Kansas City Chiefs head coach Andy Reid was right when he told ESPN the Magazine that a game plan is "where everything starts." The plan, according to Reid, depends on the coach sitting down with the quarterback to pick which plays will make it to the field that Sunday. "It's not what the coach knows but what the players know," Reid says. It's the same for you—you need more than an idea of what's going on, what's been done, and what you should do about it. You need a plan. In fact, this plan may be *required*—Medicare head, Patrick Conway, pointed out that one of the new healthcare models, called the Comprehensive Primary Care Initiative, actually requires a living, interactive plan that must be updated every visit. When you're managing your own plan, remember the acronym P.L.A.N.S. Here's how to organize your goals, tasks, and priorities:

- **P**atient Centered: The game plan has to be designed around you, your wishes and preferences, your strengths and weaknesses, and your family.
- **L**earning: You are the expert on you and your doctor is an expert on medicine. There will be a two-way exchange that will increase your doctor's familiarity with all of your symptoms and medical history in addition to all your wishes and preferences. At the same time, you will increase your knowledge of medicine and your particular medical conditions or how to improve your health. Implicit in this is learning that leads to understanding. Education and materials and mechanisms to facilitate this learning are vital to all plans.
- **A**ssignments: All good game plans have roles and assignments. This is especially important with healthcare being delivered in teams of teams. Assignments lead to accountability. Everyone on the team will have assignments including you, your doctor, nurses, and specialists.
- **N**otify: Communication is the foundation of any great team. In healthcare, information must flow across the teams of teams. Many times, this involves notifying one member of the team about a change in your situation or sometimes it is just notifying your team that you went to see another doctor. Everyone must know when to notify and close the communication gap.
- **S**uccess: In the NFL winning is the real test of a successful game plan. What is a win for you? This is where you set goals and see if you need to adjust the game plan in order to reach them.

This section of this book will look at the complexities of care in a number of settings, but no matter where you receive care or who is delivering it, the idea of these P.L.A.N.S. can guide the process. Without a game plan, you can end up reactive, always a step behind your condition. With a game plan, you can take control of your care, moving toward the goals you want instead of just running away from the medical outcomes that scare you. Keep P.L.A.N.S. in mind as you read the following chapters. But first, let's take a closer look at each step.

## Patient-Centered

In 2010 the Super Bowl broke a 27-year record for the most watched TV show in history, with 106 million viewers watching the Saints win in their first Super Bowl appearance. The previous record holder had been the final episode of M*A*S*H*, a show that embodied patient-centered care. The show was, of course, about the Korean War, and in one episode a severely wounded soldier came into the makeshift surgical theater with damage to both hands and both feet. His critical situation forced a decision to save one or the other but the patient was not able to communicate. The surgeon chose to let the patient lose his hands thinking the soldier would prefer to be able to walk. When the wounded man woke up he was horrified. He had been a concert pianist. What was the correct call in the eyes of the surgeon was incorrect from the patient-centered point of view. Of course, in this situation, the patient couldn't *express* his point of view. If you don't speak up, you might as well be the concert pianist. Healthcare is increasingly working toward patient-centered care, but in order to take advantage of this paradigm shift, you have to let healthcare know your preferences. Speak up. Ask your team to see things from your point of view. When your plan is not patient-centered, call a timeout. The issues that can and should be patient-centered range from scheduling difficulties because you work a night shift to end-of-life wishes. Make sure the Game Plan starts and ends with you.

## Learning

*Pistol strong right stack act 6 Y cross divide!* Does that make sense? How about, "The vasopressin receptor antagonist blocks reabsorption in the collecting duct correcting the hyponatremia through aquaresis"? You better believe the first one makes sense to the Arizona Cardinals offense—it's a play from their book. And the second one makes sense to doctors. But if you're not playing wide receiver for the Cardinals, you're going to need the play spelled out for you…maybe something like "Go long!" And if you're in the doctor's office, you're going to need your diagnosis and treatment instructions in plain language. The thing is, medicine has gotten so complicated that there's often no good way to say things in plain language. This means that your plan will involve learning that will in turn lead to understanding about your problem. Patients enter the healthcare system with different levels of understanding—some have PhDs and end up teaching me about the latest research on something they have been studying for years. On the other hand, I often diagnose patients with things they have never even heard of. Your doctor will start your process of learning, and should be able to direct you to more information or other sources to continue your learning. Importantly, when it comes to your medical care, learning isn't optional—it is an essential piece of your ability to collaborate on shared decisions.

One key I see that helps patients learn the information they need is the willingness to speak up when they don't understand. There is no shame in not knowing! (The same way there is no shame in not knowing how to run a play for the Arizona Cardinals.) Doctors have spent almost 30,000 hours learning medicine and there's no way you should be expected to bring the same level of understanding to the table.

But learning goes both ways. The other side of learning is the doctor's part. Your doctor has to learn everything he or she can not only to diagnose your problem today, but also to predict how it will evolve in the future and help drive the direction of your care toward your goals. Every minute detail of your headache can be important. All your prior medical and surgical problems and your family history or their medical problems can be vital to making the right diagnosis. Hopefully your doctor will create the right environment where you feel comfortable contributing to her learning, just as she contributes to yours. As the great NFL coach Bill Walsh told the *Harvard Business Journal*, "The head coach has to make it clear that he expects everyone to participate and volunteer his or her thoughts, impressions, and ideas. The goal is to create a communication channel that allows important information to get from the bottom to the top."

As part of your Health Game Plan, here are some of the things you should help your doctor learn:

- ▶ Keep track of your symptoms and then go through the list with your doctor.
- ▶ Make sure your doctor has access to your medical record, including past tests and test results.

- ▶ Talk to your parents about their medical history and then talk with your doctor about how your parents' risks influence your risks.
- ▶ Share your strengths and weakness; for instance let your doctor know if you have trouble remembering to take medications three times per day, or if you're very good at keeping track of your blood pressure with a home monitor.
- ▶ Don't be embarrassed to share your fears.
- ▶ Be honest. Don't worry about impressing or disappointing your doctor. It's better for your doctor to know you have missed medications or forgotten some of your assignments. All patients do! If you feel judged, you may need a new coach.

## Assignments

The cover of this book is the Xs and Os of a football play. Look closely and you can see that each X and O has an assignment—a specific thing they must do to ensure that the play works. In medicine, you are more like the entire team than just one X or O—instead of one assignment during a four-second play, you will have many assignments that can take place over years. But the idea of "assignments" is the same—your game plan should include the things you will do and also the things your doctor and other players on the healthcare team should do.

Doctors and nurses list their assignments on your chart or electronic medical record. They are even able to set reminders like "ask about patient's last pneumonia shot" or "remind patient to get a colonoscopy." These assignments are a doctor's to-do list, a collection of tasks that we work on throughout the day.

For you, there is a less formal process of designating assignments. And because the process is less formal, there's a higher chance of blown assignments. When a cornerback doesn't pick up the right wide receiver, the defense breaks down. If you blow an assignment, the consequences can be even worse. I know that "assignments" are also those things you had in middle school—your teacher's orders that you had to follow whether you wanted to or not. Don't take healthcare "assignments" the same way. Your doctor's assignments are an extremely important part of making sure you get the highest quality care.

Everyone is familiar with the usual assignments: fill these prescriptions, take this medication three times a day, go to physical therapy, quit smoking, eat better, and so on. Doctors can give you an assignment, but that doesn't mean you will execute it. When you make P.L.A.N.S., if an assignment doesn't feel right or you know it is impossible then it's time to revise the plan. A plan can't be written for the ideal world; it has to be written for the real world, the world in which you live. For example, a study in the *New England Journal of Medicine* showed that when costs exceed the amount that is comfortable to pay, patients will forgo important medications and treatments. If you look at your plan and see that the out-of-pocket expenses (OOPs!) will be more than you can afford, be realistic. Instead of walking away with pieces of the plan you won't follow, talk to your doctor about other options. One way to talk to your doctor about cost is by bringing it up in the context of value. You can say something like, "I would like to know the quality of outcomes and costs associated with each treatment so I can make the best value decision. With my high deductible, this will be out of my pocket!"

## Notify

In 1956 two inventors, John Campbell and George Sarles, invented the first helmet radio. The legendary Cleveland Browns coach at the time, Paul Brown, was famous for sending plays into the game with a substituted player. Knowing this, the inventors contacted Coach Brown and asked if the coach wanted to pilot the helmet radio with his quarterback, George Ratterman. Before putting the radio in his quarterback's helmet, Brown wanted to make sure it worked. He sent the inventors off to test it, which they did with Sarles walking into the woods to see how far he could go before Campbell lost the signal. Unfortunately, the local police picked up the transmissions and, thinking something suspicious was going on, arrived to arrest Sarles. It's a good thing the police officer who showed up to make the arrest was a Browns fan! The team went on to use the helmet radio until the league cottoned on and outlawed it. Now quarterbacks and one defensive player have been allowed to wear radio receivers in their helmets. It is only one way—coach to player—and it's inactivated 15 seconds before every play.

Unfortunately, this one-way communication has been the norm in healthcare, as well. Too often, doctors speak and patients are expected to listen. Modern healthcare is trying to change this. Two-way communication is critical across your teams of teams. For an obvious example, there are times when you must notify your healthcare team of a change in your condition in order to avoid serious harm. Conversely, your healthcare team has to notify you of important findings and changes in the plan as well. This is critical across the entire team, doctor to doctor, nurse to doctor, doctor to nurse, doctor to specialist, and all the other combinations. As I have seen too many times, failure in this system of notifications can have devastating consequences.

## Success

Pat Kirwan, the former Jets defensive coach and salary cap expert, hit the nail on the head when he told me, "In the NFL it is easy to see who won. Winning is the goal. In healthcare, it is not that easy." You may have the same condition, the same history, the same symptoms as another person, but your goals can be completely different. For you and this other patient, "success" would have very different meanings.

Great Health Game Plans need to define what is "winning" from a patient's perspective. This is one of the basic tenets of the push toward what medicine calls "patient-centered care." The win or achieving that goal can be as simple as sitting up without pain or as ambitious as running a marathon, as basic as seeing your children without being zonked on pain medication, or as complex as being able to play your favorite song on your guitar. Some wins are obvious—a cure for cancer or successful gallbladder removal without any complications. Some are just numbers—blood pressure at the right target or cholesterol in the correct range. But many successes are much more subjective depending on what is important to the patient.

One reason you want to define "success" in your health game plan is that without a measure of success you won't know if you have succeeded. If you realize you have not met success, you can adjust so that you can improve. In this way, the cycle of a health game plan is much like an NFL game plan. At some point, you review the film to see how you did.

Then you adjust the plan to improve, passing through this cycle as many times as you need to reach your goals. Like an NFL game, you can make adjustments from season to season, game to game, half to half, or in the middle of a play.

Finally, defining success lets you celebrate when you reach it. High five or fist bump your doctor or healthcare team when your results come back better. We are so busy with the grind and paperwork of medicine that I think we don't celebrate the successes enough. I know I don't. Helping patients achieve their goals is why most of us doctors went into the field of medicine in the first place.

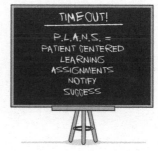

# CHAPTER 14:
## Maximizing Home-Field Advantage in the Outpatient Setting

I knew a big man once. He looked down on just about everyone, but never felt above. From an early age he earned the favor of his teachers by erasing the top of the black board or hanging the highest holiday decoration. Everyone knew him, even people he never met. Despite his size even the most conversation-adverse frequent fliers, armed with headphones and e-books, would end up exchanging pleasantries.

As a teacher, he also loved kids. He had a big heart, seeing hopeful futures where others saw troubled headaches. He never gave up on kids, even those who gave up on themselves. He always knew what was going on, a human surveillance camera perched high in the sky.

If parents are unsung heroes, stepparents are just as unsung. I know because that's how I met this man. He was my children's stepfather, my ex-wife's husband. He became the chauffeur of the family: football practice, musical theater, dance, voice, surfing…oh! and he was the assistant dean of the best high school in the county, in his spare time. Together we maneuvered a schedule matched only by Grand Central: drop off Emily at 1:25 pm, pickup 3:30 pm; next pick up Josh at 3:45 pm and CC needs to be at dance at 4:30 pm, and so it went until 11:00 at night. Hence my surprise one evening when I picked up my children and my ex-wife was there instead.

This particular night her face was taut with concern, "Can I ask you about my husband? I'm worried about him," she said. I hugged the girls but noting the mom-and-dad-need-to talk body language, they jumped into my car waging their perennial fight over shotgun. My ex-wife began to tell me about the swelling in his legs and feet before saying, "He is short of breath and I know he is heavier than he should be, plus he is always tired. All summer he's been ignoring my pleas to see a doctor. He is finally going tomorrow though." I told her that was the right thing to do. I told her that my first concern would be about his heart.

We all knew the doctor—the doctor's children went to the school where my ex-wife's husband was assistant principal and they had worked together on community projects. But when he went to the doctor's office the next day, he saw a nurse practitioner instead. He told her about the pain in his chest that was worse last night and how he just did not feel like himself. She asked questions and did an exam, then ordered blood tests, an X-ray and an EKG. Then he waited. And waited. And waited. Multiple times throughout the day he called the family with updates, with the news that his heart enzymes were high but all else was okay and so they were repeating the heart enzyme test. For the rest of the day until they were about to close there was confusion on the enzyme results, which had, by that point, been repeated multiple times. He wondered if he should just go to the hospital.

Finally, the nurse practitioner bolted back into the room. "It is just reflux. Take this medicine. We want you to take a stress test next week, but we can arrange that. The doctor doesn't think the first blood test was correct. The others are lower," she said. Relieved, but confused, he didn't argue. He trusted his doctor and hurried out of the office as it closed.

My son, hearing of the doctor's visit, decided to stop by the house to check in on him. After dinner, he seemed okay, but he asked my son, "Would reflux cause this kind of chest pain?" My son didn't know the answer, but was relieved that he seemed to be okay. He went outside to talk to his mother.

After about 20 minutes they came back in but he was no longer sitting in his chair. Walking around the couch my ex-wife screamed, "Oh my God!" He was face down on the floor, not moving, breathing, or responding. They screamed and pounded on his back but there was nothing; they struggled to turn his motionless body over. He was not breathing and had no pulse. While my son called 911, my ex-wife began CPR. Using more and more pressure, screaming his name, my son was horrified to hear a rib crack, a sound no child should hear. After an eternity, the paramedics arrived and so did my other son. Trying to keep their mother calm they did everything possible to save his life—shocking, medication, and oxygen.

The lead paramedic finally came outside. "I am sorry," he said, "we did everything we could but he is gone."

According to a study by Hardeep Singh, MD, MPH, nationally recognized patient safety expert at the Baylor School of Medicine, one-in-twenty outpatients are misdiagnosed. I sat down with Dr. Singh at his office in Houston where he shared his insights about this under-recognized problem of outpatient misdiagnosis.

The ACA and other forces are moving healthcare away from big hospital settings and into the offices of your primary care physician or nurse practitioner. Surgeries previously done in a hospital with a five-day stay are now being done in a free-standing surgery center with patients going home the same day. Certain blood clots that used to buy you a stay in the hospital are being treated at home. Freestanding Emergency rooms now can keep you overnight just for observation and testing and send you home in 14 hours, avoiding the hospital. While outpatient visits climb, hospital admissions continue to fall every year, showing the shift toward less specialized levels of care.

This shift can mean less expense and less headache. It can also mean that your care is handled in a setting with fewer experts and fewer resources. Like my ex-wife's husband, this can lead to misdiagnosis. I don't want to vilify doctors or healthcare teams in outpatient settings. Making a correct medical diagnosis can be simple and obvious, or it can be the most elusive and challenging aspect of being a doctor. Doctors spend years studying thousands of hours to even start to become good at this process. I have made some wrong diagnoses and have made others later than I would have liked. In part, that's because despite our technological, scientific, and cultural advances in medicine, medical diagnosis remains both an art and a science.

Once as a chief resident I remember speaking to a room full of scared interns about to take care of real patients as practicing doctors for the first time. My most important advice for them was that admitting when they didn't know some-thing was more important than displaying what they knew. I used to draw a circle and say it is not the size of your circle of knowledge but knowing the edge of the circle that will keep patients safe. Despite awareness and training, keeping in mind the limits of this circle of knowledge remains desperately diffi-cult for physicians.

Dr. Singh showed this in a study that has since become famous. He gave 118 practicing physicians two cases, one easy and one hard. In addition to asking the doctors to diagnose both cases, he asked them to rate their confidence in each diagnosis. The doctors correctly diagnosed the easy case only 60 percent of the time and only six percent were correct on the difficult case. Now "easy" and "difficult" are subjective categories and so we could argue that 60 percent and six percent are not especially meaningful representations of how often doctors are likely to succeed in other "easy" and "diffi-cult" cases. But here's the important number: On the easier cases, doctors scored their confidence as 7.2 on a 1–10 scale; on these more difficult cases that only about 1-in-20 doctors got correct, their confidence was *only slightly lower* at 6.4 on this scale. Results were published in the November 2013 issue of *JAMA*. Even when doctors were wrong, they were confident that they were right.

This is not a book for doctors but for you. I want to help you understand how to be the safety for your healthcare team, which can be especially important outside the wrap-around services of a hospital. The outpatient setting is your home turf—it is your own handcrafted team of doctors and tends to take place in the settings you know best. This means that the outpatient setting can offer tremendous home field advantage...if you know how to take advantage of it. But it also means you can be blindsided.

In 1960, the Eagles played the Giants at Yankee Stadium. With the Eagles winning 17-10 late in the game, Frank Gifford caught a pass across the middle and Chuck Bednarik hit him so hard it knocked him up into the air and it snapped his head back violently against the hard turf. Gifford never saw it coming. He was knocked out and carried off the field. Gifford would miss the rest of the season and all of the next. This is what happens when you're blindsided.

The first step to ensuring you are not blindsided on your home turf is ensuring that you don't switch teams every year! NFL teams use dramatically different systems and so a player that goes from one to another has to learn a whole new system. The plays are different not to mention the formations and the signals. The team needs to learn the player too. The same is true in healthcare—going to many offices means that you will have to know many systems. Sticking with one home team is a good lesson not just for your use of primary care, but across your entire health system. The more integrated or "tightly packed" is your system, the more easily you will be able to manage your care within it.

Kaiser Permanente is the classic example. If Kaiser is your insurance and your PCP and your specialists and your hospital, you can get home-field advantage for your entire care experience. Your doctor can text the lab and your records will all be on the same system available for everyone to see. Their scheduling system and their email and their electronic medical record will all be the same and you only have to get to know one. This integration can make coordinating your care much easier, helping you get the most from your outpatient experience.

The reason that Kaiser can wrap patients in home-field advantage is that Kaiser built its team by adding all the pieces. Other health systems are following suit—hospitals have started their own insurance plans, they have bought PCP and specialist practices, and usually already have lab and imaging facilities. From another side of the coin, insurance companies are buying and hiring PCPs and specialists and even buying urgent cares and hospitals. The ACA disallowed physicians or physician-groups from owning hospitals, but many were grandfathered in, meaning that doctors, too, are making systems that offer more home-field advantage.

What is the downside? Sometimes these integrated health-care systems offer ease at the expense of choice. You may not like one member of the team. You like the PCP but not their specialists. You like the hospital but not their insurance plan. You like their specialists but don't like their PCPs.

Another way to maximize home field advantage is by playing as many home games as possible. Outpatient care has a rhythm. For some of you who are healthy you might see your PCP once a year, if that. Your rhythm is like an entire offseason between visits. But, in my opinion, the pros of more frequent checkups outweigh the cons—healthcare is a series of touch points, some known and some unknown, and it is always good to sit down at least once a year with your head coach and go over your goals and observations and fears even if you are healthy. Your relationship with your head coach is a vital relationship that takes time and communication to lead to trust. I have saved lives by picking up small things in my office during a routine exam. And making this connection with your PCP plugs you into the system. It gives you a team that has your records and if a problem arises at least you have a place to start. As we will discuss in later chapters, that does not mean you should always go there for every problem, but you will have a better chance of catching important health changes if your doctor has seen you consistently before these changes took place.

Then, of course, is the huge problem of misdiagnosis. If my ex-wife's husband had had a correct diagnosis, he might still be alive. Getting a correct diagnosis can be especially important in the outpatient setting because you will be sent home to follow through with your treatment—if the diagnosis is wrong, you won't be sticking around in a setting where doctors can catch and fix this error. Here are things you can do to maximize your chances of leaving an outpatient visit with a game plan that addresses the correct game—Dr. Singh offers numbers 1–3 and the rest in this list are from my experience of patients, diagnosis and safety.

## 1. Get Your History Right

For six months, a patient I knew (but was not my own!) underwent chemotherapy to treat what her team diagnosed as early-stage lung cancer. During her treatment and follow-up visits, she told her nurse practitioner and nursing team that she had back pain, but explained that she had had this pain for quite some time, even before she was diagnosed with lung cancer. Because the team was focused on her cancer, they chose not to explore this symptom. Months went by. Finally, this patient went to an orthopedic doctor to look at how they might treat this muscle- or bone-related pain and as part of the diagnostic process, the orthopedist ordered a spine CT. In her spine, they found multiple tumors that were metastatic from her lung. Her lung cancer was not early stage. It was stage four. I am sharing this not to blame the doctors that treated this patient but to show how a small bit of information not completely understood by the team and not shared among the team can lead to missed or delayed diagnoses.

The story you tell your doctor is critical to the diagnosis. Doctors know this—studies have shown almost 80 percent of a diagnosis comes from what you tell your doctor and from the statistics of your initial physical exam. Of course, doctors have a role in this story by asking the right questions. You have a role too: You need to prepare to tell your story. List the history of your symptoms and prepare to deliver this history to your doctor. I cannot stress enough the importance of detailing the changes in your health that you have experienced—the things that are getting worse, things that are different. If this patient's P.A. had asked if her pain was different than her usual back pain or if the patient had volunteered this information, they might have made changes sooner in her treatment that could have affected the trajectory of her cancer. Like the NFL where information is gathered and used obsessively, you can never say too much or bring too much information to the table.

## 2. Your Doctor's Second Opinion

One of the takeaways from Dr. Singh and his study was that doctors should offer their own second opinion. He said that patients can ask, *"What else could it be?"* to encourage their doctors to consider other possibilities. This isn't out of the ordinary. All doctors are taught something called a "differential diagnosis," which is a fancy term for making a list of things that could be causing your problem, one of which hopefully is your correct diagnosis. Sometimes this list is small and other times it can be very long. There are things on the list that can be deadly and others that will go away on their own. Amazingly, Dr. Singh shared that when his team reviewed patient charts as part of another study, this differential diagnosis was absent more than half the time! In one day, a doctor might see thirty patients with simple colds, but doctors still have to keep their heads in the game so they don't miss that one patient whose "cold" is actually a life-threatening throat infection.

In my experience, it's good for doctors and patients to discuss these possibilities and the likelihood that any one of them is the real problem (or problems). Doctors and patients should also discuss a plan to eliminate some of the possibilities to get to the answer. If possible, it's also good for the other members of your healthcare team to participate in this conversation. Verbalizing the process of differential diagnosis can trigger an important insight for you, your doctor, or other team members. Think of it like the HBO show *Hard Knocks*, which takes place inside NFL training camps. Often the program shows coaches sitting in meetings with or without players, discussing their game plan. You can see decisions being made collaboratively with everyone sharing not just their opinions but their thought processes as well. As a patient, you can encourage this collaborative "talking through" of all the possible options.

## 3. No News Is Not Always Good News

Dr. Singh points out that patients often think that no news is good news—if they don't hear back from their doctor, then everything must be fine. Unfortunately, that's not always the case and if you don't hear back from your doctor, it can be your job to follow up. Don't have test results? Didn't hear back from your PCP office? Keep pressing until you have answers. Again, you shouldn't have to do this and it isn't your role, but that doesn't take away from the fact that following up until you get answers may be the most important thing you do for your diagnosis.

This lack of follow-up communication even happened to me, with a doctor I know well! When I turned 50, I, of course, had the pleasure of my first colonoscopy and I chose a gastroenterologist I had worked with many times. During the procedure the team found some polyps that were biopsied. Then I waited...and waited...and never heard back about the biopsy results. I had to press them and finally track down the results myself. Luckily everything was fine, but what if I were not so fortunate? What if these polyps were cancerous? Even knowing these polyps were non-cancerous, the result changed my screening recommendation to five years rather than ten. What if I thought no news was good news and came back ten years later to discover that new, more dangerous polyps had started to grow?

## 4. Ask Why

Remember when you encouraged your children to be curious until they drove you crazy with the question *why*? Now it's your turn. Drive your healthcare team crazy by always asking *why*. Why do I need this test? Why do you think this is a problem with my heart? Why do you recommend surgery or this procedure? Why am I taking this medicine? This helps drive communication and lessens the chance of misunderstanding. Doctors are supposed to have this "why" in their heads, but curating this understanding yourself allows you to collaborate on your diagnosis and potentially help to catch misdiagnoses and other errors yourself. Why not ask why?

## 5. Trust Your Gut

My children's stepfather knew in his gut something was not right with his diagnosis of reflux and even spoke with my son about it just before he died. His wife heard his misgivings and even told him to go to the ER. When you feel like something is wrong, there very well may be something wrong. Call a timeout! Good doctors and coaches listen to their patients. If your arm pain is so severe that the diagnosis of a simple sprain seems incorrect, speak up. If you have the worst headache you've ever had and know it's more than "just a migraine," speak up. If the doctor's diagnosis just doesn't seem to fit your experience, speak up. You are part of the team. Good doctors will listen and explain their thoughts. It's possible that they will open their mind to other possibilities.

## 6. If Your Treatment Is Not Working, Speak Up

This sounds simple, but many patients remain silent in their suffering. If you are not responding to your prescribed treatment, it's a good time to rethink the diagnosis. Speak up! Your doctor should tell you when you should expect to see improvement. When you tell your doctor that you're not, in fact, improving, it's his or her job to listen and respect the possibility that treatment has been misdirected.

## 7. Like an NFL Receiver, Hands Are Important

If your doctor doesn't physically examine you, that's a warning sign. My godfather, also a doctor, recently told me about a patient who was seen for pain in his collarbone. Without even pressing on the collarbone, the doctor assumed it was a fracture but when an X-ray was negative, the doctor downgraded the diagnosis to a sprain. When my godfather saw him, the patient had a fever and when he pushed on the spot that hurt, he felt an enlarged spot. When my godfather sent the patient to the hospital, they found an abscess in his collarbone where it meets the breastbone. Had the first doctor used his hands, he would have found the abscess right away.

## 8. When in Doubt, Get a Second Opinion

Another set of eyes and a fresh brain never hurt. A good doctor will never be offended and might even encourage you to get a second opinion. Medicine is so complex that nobody knows it all, and if someone professes to know it all, run!

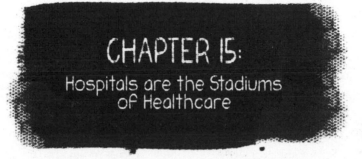

# CHAPTER 15:
## Hospitals are the Stadiums of Healthcare

Throughout my more than 20-year career I have spent more than 1,000 nights in hospitals. As a doctor, that is. Almost as enlightening were the 10 nights I spent at my wife's side during her hospitalization. I already wrote about how a surgeon announced to her room full of guests on the way out the door, "Oh, by the way your X-ray has a lung nodule, we will need to do a CAT scan." And how he didn't order it until I reminded him: "Oh, yeah, I forgot," he said almost laughing, only to have it show more than five blood clots in my wife's lungs that could have been fatal. However, the shortcomings of one doctor in this hospital system are not what I want to focus on. No, I want to talk about our experience.

During my wife's stay every nurse and doctor (except one) was beyond reproach. Some knew I was a doctor but I knew none of the doctors or nurses as I had never worked in this hospital. I also watched them interact with other patients and families and they were just as excellent. The nurses in particular communicated well and the team was very coordinated. They were extremely responsive to our requests to see test results and other information.

The patient's ambassador dogs helped my wife's pain. They made the five steps to the bathroom easier. That walk would have seemed like running a marathon without the dogs. It was a Catholic hospital and, dressed in black, the priest brought surprising comfort during his visits too. In fact, I used to wear black as a doctor—some patients used to joke that I looked like Johnny Cash and I remember once a patient thought I looked like Atlanta Falcons coach, Jerry Glanville, who famously dressed in all black (and left tickets for Elvis at the will-call booth, even a decade after Elvis's death). My all-black days ended when a patient mistook me as a mortician. I try not to wear black anymore.

In any case, during my wife's stay, she was able to order her food as if calling for room service, 24 hours a day on her television, which was also a computer with instant online access. All her patient education was ready on her TV at her fingertips. She could read or watch videos about her colon surgery or her blood clots. As a reminder, doctors even asked about her health screening, like her last mammogram.

A patient experience representative came daily to ask if there was anything else we needed. The entire hospital was brand new and designed like a theme park with separate elevators for transporting patients and entire hallways for the staff hidden to the public. From the moment she was rushed to the emergency room with a dying colon until the day she got in the car to go home, the support and care was fantastic. It was the best of teams and facilities.

I say all this because, for me, it was a unique view from the patient perspective on a system I see every day. According to business and management guru Peter Drucker, hospitals are "the most complex human organization ever devised." That's true...when they *work*. But now that hospitals are becoming insurance companies and doctors' practices and responsible for thousands of patients outside the hospital, I would call them the most complex human disorganizations ever devised!

You can think about hospitals as the stadiums of healthcare, their towers framing city skylines like coliseums of care. Billboards line highways extolling their greatest victories and highlighting their connections to the community. Walk into a hospital atrium and you can see its "championship banners" bragging about rankings and accomplishments, the faces of star players and coaches beaming from posters. If you think that hospitals becoming like stadiums is a new thing, consider this: Early hospitals actually had amphitheaters where crowds of medical students watched the great surgeons perform at the top of their game.

Hospitals share another important similarity with NFL stadiums: You own them. Of 32 NFL teams, one stadium is privately owned, three are owned by teams, and one is shared between the team and private owners. The rest are publicly owned. Almost the same ownership numbers are true of hospitals. There are approximately 32 million admissions a year to public hospitals and only 2 million to private ones. This means that neither hospitals nor NFL stadiums are "ivory towers" set apart from the rest of the world. NFL stadiums have to benefit the cities that pay to build them; hospitals have to benefit the communities that own them. In fact, current laws require them to survey their impact on their communities to make sure they derive the benefit for their nonprofit and publicly owned status.

Hospitals deliver healthcare's greatest wins, from heart transplants to face transplants, from laparoscopic surgery to stereotactic brain biopsies, while patients are awake. It is in hospitals that trauma victims survive against all odds and cancer patients are cured with bone marrow transplants. In hospitals, babies born at 21 weeks have survived their premature entrance into the world. Hospitals are the best of what we can accomplish with science and compassion. That is, most of the time. They can also be unintentionally dangerous, putting their already at-risk patients at even more risk.

Here is something vitally important across all aspects of healthcare and health insurance: The more you know, the safer you will be. Getting the most value with the least risk from your time in the hospital starts with knowing how the hospital works. Let's take a look now.

## Getting Into the Stadium

For better or for worse, a hospital's "main gate" is the ER. Eighty-five percent of the patients in a hospital came in through the ER. Like a stadium's main gate, it may have taken a long wait amid significant chaos to get in. That said, there are other ways to enter the hospital. Just as many NFL stadiums have clubs with private entrances, some patients enter the hospital without having to navigate the ER. If you are scheduled to have surgery, you will go to an office and then to a special pre-op area where your team will get you ready for surgery. If you are having a baby (unless you are literally *having* a baby) you will check in at the OB area. Finally, some of you will be sent to the hospital by your doctor who has called ahead to arrange a bed—this is called a direct admission. You usually need to go to the admissions office first and then you can go to a hospital room, avoiding the ER. A few of you will go from one hospital directly to another, this is called a **transfer**. With a transfer, sometimes you will have to make a stop in the ER but in most cases, you will go straight to your hospital room.

## Are You in the Game or on the Sidelines? (OOPs! Alert!)

On average, patients who are admitted through the ER will stay four days as inpatients. Others who are treated in the ER but who are well enough to be sent home are outpatients. Somewhere in between outpatient and inpatient status is *observation*. Medicare created this status called "Observation" for patients that didn't really meet criteria for hospital admission but whose conditions were serious enough to make going home inappropriate. At first, observation status was used while monitoring or clarifying the diagnosis, for example while waiting on test results. During this time, the team will be expediting your tests and your doctors may see you more frequently. If a hospital isn't reimbursed at a higher rate for this specialized care, it can lead to a TEAM–me conflict in which it's best for you to stay, but best for the hospital to get you out the door quickly. On the other hand, admitting you to the hospital can lead to another TEAM–me conflict in which you need to stay, but your *insurance* company doesn't want to pay for expensive hospital care and so wants you out the door as quickly as possible. Observation status was meant to split the difference, reimbursing hospitals for these patients who use more than ER services but less than the services of the full hospital.

The problem—and what you need to be aware of—is that technically when you are in observation status in the hospital you are actually an outpatient. So your co-pays are not managed the way they would be if you were fully admitted. This catches many patients by surprise. For example, Medicare makes you responsible for 20 percent of the bill and requires that you pay the cost of your medications administered while in observation status. Supplemental or "gap" insurance covers many of these OOPs! expenses but not everyone has this protection. Here's another catch: If you are admitted to a hospital and are then transferred to a skilled nursing home or rehabilitation center, chances are your insurance will be required to cover this additional treatment. (Medicare covers skilled care after three days of hospital care with *admission* status.) However, if you are transferred to one of these care facilities from "observation," you can end up responsible for the entire bill! I have seen patients face $40,000 bills from this scenario. If you are in observation status and are switched to admission status, your time in observation does not count towards Medicare's required three-day stay.

In 2015, Congress passed legislation requiring hospitals to notify you when you are in observation status for more than 24 hours but to date this requirement has not really been operationalized. Just remember: Always ask if you are admitted or in observation status and what this will mean for your part of the bill. In many cases, this observation status lets insurer and hospital come to a fair middle ground between reimbursement levels for outpatient and

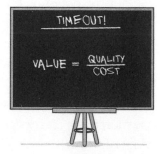

inpatient statuses, and thus lets you stay a bit longer where doctors can watch your condition. But it also has the potential to influence your bottom line, sticking you with more of the bill. If you are in Observation status and stay longer than 24 hours make sure to ask if your status has changed and how that will affect your bill. When in doubt, call your health insurance to make sure everyone is on the same page.

## Hospitalists Are Interim Head Coaches

Colts head coach Chuck Pagano was hospitalized for much of the 2012 season, fighting leukemia. During that time, offensive coach Bruce Arians took the reins as interim head coach. Pagano tried to keep calling the shots. According to articles, Pagano would call Arians from his hospital bed giving advice and guidance from a distance. The day-to-day coaching, however, was in Bruce Arians' hands. When he was cleared to return home Coach Pagano resumed the reins.

The relationship between head coach Chuck Pagano and interim head coach Bruce Arians is like the relationship between your primary care provider and the hospitalist who oversees your inpatient care. Your primary care physician is your head coach in the outpatient setting. A hospitalist becomes your interim head coach when you are admitted.

Hospitalists are different than primary care providers. They have expertise in hospital-based care and in improving the value of care in that setting. They think in terms of treating the entire population of patients at the hospital and not just about how to treat you. For example, a hospitalist thinks of the best way to treat pneumonia not just for you but for all patients with pneumonia. In addition to keeping in mind the needs of the all the sick people in the hospital, an old boss of mine, Dr. Adam Singer, was fond of calling the hospital itself another patient—one that a hospitalist needs to treat in addition to their actual patients.

The hospitalist movement has migrated to specialties as well, including pediatrics, OB and surgery. This means these doctors only practice in the setting of their hospital—so don't be surprised to see them!

I am not only a hospitalist, but am the National Medical Director for Team Health/IPC, one of the largest integrated healthcare providers in the U.S. We have more than 19,000 doctors in more than 30 states. This is to say that I might be a little bit biased toward the importance of hospitalists. But unless your PCP regularly goes to the hospital to see patients, a good hospitalist is a priority. It's like having a good interim head coach. A hospitalist may consult with other specialists but he or she serves the same coordinating role as do PCPs outside the hospital.

## Specialists in the Hospital

When you go to an ER, specialists are assigned or volunteer to be on call to consult on your case or delivery specialty care. This means, for example, that if you break your hip and need surgery you will be assigned the orthopedist who is on call at that time. (That is, unless you already have a relationship with an orthopedist, in which case the ER would bring your orthopedist into the team.) On the other hand, if you fall while you are in the hospital and break your hip, your hospitalist or PCP is free to refer you to the orthopedist of their choice— your own orthopedist if you have one, or a new orthopedist if you don't. What does this mean to you? If you already have a specialist make sure everyone on your hospital team knows so they can use your specialist if possible.

There are even times when your specialist will be your head coach. This is most often the case when you go into the hospital for a planned surgery. Let's say you have an elective or planned hip replacement. Your orthopedist will be the head coach and a hospitalist or PCP will only be called in to help. Yes, this is confusing! If you don't understand who is on your hospital team, call a timeout! Ask, ask, ask who everyone is and what is their role on the team.

## Your Hospital Schedule

While John Gruden was the head coach of the Tampa Bay Buccaneers he was famous for getting up every morning at 3:17 am. The timing of your doctor visits in the hospital, however, can be much less predictable. Like a good coach, your doctor will take their entire team of patients into account when planning their day. You could be first or you could be last. Some of the other aspects of the hospital routine are as-possible as well, while some are scheduled. When you are first admitted, ask about the schedule and ask which tasks you can expect at certain times and which will happen whenever the staff gets to it. Here are many of the check-ins, checkups and other visits and tasks you should expect during your hospital stay:

## SCHEDULED

- ▶ Blood draws
- ▶ Medications—likely on a 4-, 6-, 8-, 12-, or 24-hour schedule
- ▶ The end of your nurse's shift (every 8 or 12 hours)

- Planned procedures and tests
- Sometimes team rounds
- Meals (though some hospitals allow you to order at your leisure)
- Visiting hours
- Cafeteria hours for visitors
- Office hours for administrative services and pharmacy

## UNSCHEDULED

- Doctor or team rounds (check-ins with your coaching staff)
- Physical therapy and other rehabilitative services
- Non-scheduled surgeries, tests, or procedures
- Transfers from one unit to another in the hospital including from the ER to your hospital bed
- Time of discharge
- Communication between members of your healthcare team
- Lab and other test results including when tests have been read by the right doctors

## The White Board

I consider the large white board in most hospital rooms as the living patient chart for the healthcare team, designed to keep everyone informed and on the same page. Just as the NFL has replaced sideline white boards with tablets, some hospitals now use a room's flat-screen TV for this purpose. That said, some hospitals that have tried to replace the white board with technology are going back—nothing is as simple as writing on a wall-mounted board for all to see. Your hospital room white board is where your coaches draw up the plays that become your care. Here are key things it should have:

- ▶ All the key members of the team including your doctors and nurses
- ▶ Your game plan for the day
- ▶ Important goals
- ▶ Projected discharge date and key milestones
- ▶ Personal information including your nickname (if any) and family member contact info
- ▶ Any big medical red flags like allergies or special needs
- ▶ Any risks like falling that everyone on the team should know about
- ▶ Dietary timing and restrictions
- ▶ Patient education—you'd be surprised how often doctors end up drawing on the white board to help explain a patient's condition!
- ▶ Questions—you or your visitors can write important questions on the whiteboard. If there's anything specific you want to accomplish that day, write it on the board! This can help you hold your team responsible for helping you achieve your goals.

## Nurses Are the Trainers

NFL doctors set the game plans for players' health while it's the trainers who execute the plan. Nurses are the trainers of the hospital. I cannot overemphasize how important nurses are to your care. In addition to being "high touch"—meaning that of all hospital staff, nurses will spend the most time with you—they are also essential conduits of information to your doctor or specialists. A nurse can save your life by picking up vital changes in your condition. However, communication breakdown between you and your nurse or between your nurse and the rest of the team can also put you at risk. If you can't work with your nurse to solve conflicts that arise, talk to another nurse in the day's rotation or even their boss, the head nurse. Sometimes nurses (like anyone) will resent this step but remember that your care comes first. If you feel that your care is being jeopardized by conflict or bad communication with your nurse, call a timeout and speak up.

## Transitioning from the Hospital to Home

First a quick note about the mechanics of discharge: Once you're admitted to a hospital, you can't leave until your hospitalist or PCP signs your discharge papers. Of course, you can leave Against Medical Advice, or AMA, but that has both legal and financial consequences. A more common problem in this transition between the hospital and home is a breakdown between the plays you practice and the plays you execute on game day. See, in many ways your time in the hospital is only practice for how you live your life after discharge. From the moment you roll in the door you should be working towards getting home safely and then not coming back. In a hospital's physical therapy, for example, you will practice climbing stairs to simulate what you will face at home. There are many more challenges you will face at home, some of which the hospital team may never guess or might overlook. Think about all these things you will need to do when you get home and then talk to your hospital team about how you can practice them before you leave. If a patient has to perform ongoing medical self-care at home, I often ask him or her to show me exactly how they will do it before they leave the hospital—I have them show me how they use their inhaler or I watch them give themselves a shot. If your doctor doesn't ask to see you do these things, ask your doctor to watch. Take advantage of your coaches' training while they are available to you. In addition to your doctors and specialists, most hospitals have educators for diabetes or breathing problems or mental health and social issues. Now, in the hospital, is the time to take advantage of these services that can help you perform at home when it matters most.

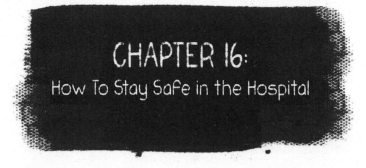

# CHAPTER 16:
## How To Stay Safe in the Hospital

"It's just a rash, what's the big deal?" Tim said to his wife, Susan. "A rash ain't gonna kill nobody."

Susan, knowing her husband would have to be near death to see a doctor, grew increasingly worried. The rash was making a steady climb up Tim's leg. Then came the fever, untouched by Acetaminophen. When he could no longer get out of bed, she became frightened. Susan called 911 and Tim was rushed to the emergency room.

After waiting for six hours, Tim finally saw the ER doctor. He was quickly diagnosed with cellulitis, a skin infection. Given his high white blood cell count and fever he was admitted for I.V. antibiotics. Susan felt relieved that she had made the right call.

The next morning my partner signed Tim out to my care. Simple case of cellulitis, on I.V. antibiotics, I was told—he should go home today. Downing a quick cup of coffee, I looked over Tim's labs. He had some baby white blood cells, which were quite high and continuing to rise, not uncommon for infection.

When I talked with Tim he related weeks of fatigue before his rash and fever, not quite consistent with cellulitis. I went through my thoughts letting the team know I was not convinced his symptoms were due to a simple infection. The next day, James's white-blood-cell count had doubled, confirming my suspicions. We have a saying in the hospital: the nicer you are, the greater the chance that you will have cancer. Susan and Tim were classic proof. A bone marrow test confirmed the diagnosis: acute leukemia.

When you are about to turn a young couple's world upside down, the walk is never long or short enough. As a doctor, you let the pain close but not inside the thin protective shell that allows you to see the rest of your patients that day. And that night your kids' hugs last just a little longer.

"How can you have cancer in your blood?" Susan cried loud enough to startle the woman delivering the patients' food.

I explained that Tim needed treatment immediately. "Tim is young and healthy, and we feel he has a chance for a cure," was all Susan heard that day.

Chemotherapy is the ultimate oxymoron. It kills your cells so that you can live—if all goes according to plan, it's a lifesaving chemical poison that kills more cancer cells than healthy cells. Susan never left Tim's side through the nausea and sweats that come with treatment, tending to his every need. She became alarmed when he spat blood after he brushed his teeth, his platelets that help blood clot low from the chemotherapy.

That night Tim had a sudden headache. Pain medication didn't touch it. Susan became more frantic especially when the nurse wrote it off as a migraine. *Tim has never had a migraine before*, she thought. Scared, Susan again pressed the nurse to call the doctor. The nurse did not.

Suddenly, Tim's eyes rolled back in his head, and he started to shake uncontrollably. The nurse called a rapid response, and other nurses and staff rushed in. Tim was clearly having a seizure. He shook violently, flopping around in his bed like a catfish out of water and hitting his head on the railing. A mass of people rushed Susan out of the room as her screams woke the entire floor.

She never spoke to her husband again.

I was not on call that night but the next morning, my partner said, "Oh yeah, one of your patients died. He had a massive bleed in his brain. He died in the CAT scan."

I pressed him for details. "His platelets were low, but we were following them. What happened? Did the nurse call you?" I asked.

"No, not until he was gone."

I had to talk to his wife that morning as she cried in the family waiting room. She was inconsolable, and I don't blame her. She told me she asked the nurse to call, she knew in her gut that something wasn't right. By the time the nurse took her seriously, it was too late.

I reported this case to the head nurse, and she acknowledged that his platelets, although not critically low, should have been considered when the nurse made the diagnosis of migraine headache—just like the inability of blood to clot after brushing his teeth, low platelets could magnify the impact of any little bleed, especially in the brain. This was not a cancer floor. Cancer nurses are much more aware of complications such as bleeding in the brain due to low platelets. A nurse on a cancer floor might not have brushed off a headache of that severity.

Here's the important question for this chapter: Is this a medical error?

Maybe surprisingly, health safety researchers might not think so. Based on the diagnosis and symptoms, it wasn't negligent for the nurse to think that Tim's headache was a migraine, maybe caused by chemotherapy. Still, it is clear that critical information was not shared with the team, namely the doctor. I have seen just as many examples where the doctor is notified but doesn't respond fast enough or in an aggressive enough manner.

I chose this case to make sure that you realize what might be the most important factor in keeping yourself and your family safe in the hospital: You are the MVP of the team. If you ever feel you are not being heard or there is a lack of response, call a timeout. Take it up the chain and ask for the chief medical officer of the hospital if you have to. It is better to over-respond than to under-respond when you feel like something isn't right.

The alternative is dangerous. In fact, you are more likely to be harmed in a hospital than an NFL player is to be hurt on any given Sunday. Yes, according to data from 10 North Carolina hospitals about 25 percent of patients are harmed during their hospital stay, with 63 percent of these harmful errors being preventable. More recent studies show about a third of all patients who visit rehabilitative hospitals or skilled nursing facilities are harmed during their stays as well.

How big of a problem is hospital error? Whenever the media picks up on medical error, hospitals and doctors tend to call it hyperbole that inaccurately overstates the problem.

They say it only stirs up fear and is meant to get a headline. I am sure doctors and hospitals will challenge this statement, although none of the safety experts I spoke with doubted this claim. In fact, on the other side, safety experts typically say the numbers underestimate the enormity of the problem. They say news reports are needed to drive awareness about medical error so that meaningful action to prevent deaths occurs with a sense of urgency. Dr. John T. James has a handle on the real scale of medical errors. After his own son died due to a medical error in 2002, James, a NASA toxicologist, studied premature deaths associated with preventable harm to patients. His number is published in the *Journal of Patient Safety*: 400,000. James found that 400,000 patients die every year due to causes that could have been prevented.

Here is the conclusion of his paper:

"The epidemic of patient harm in hospitals must be taken more seriously if it is to be curtailed. Fully engaging patients and their advocates during hospital care, systematically seeking the patients' voice in identifying harms, transparent accountability for harm, and intentional correction of root causes of harm will be necessary to accomplish this goal."

After reading his paper and visiting his website, I reached out to Dr. James and he graciously invited me to meet him at his home. In the comfort of his living room the agony of his lost son resurfaced as he took me back to those tragic days.

"The pain always pours back in when I talk about it," he said through tears. Although he asked me not to retell the full details of his son's story, the basic outline is that his son died from a combination of mistakes centering on a low potassium level that was not replaced adequately. Now he has dedicated his life to ensuring no other patients and family members suffer in the same way.

Now years after the publication of his initial study, James has come to the conclusion that we regularly underestimate the number and impact of medical errors on patients' lives. Most errors are small and don't inflict serious harm. Often errors are caught just in time, right before they could have been catastrophic, like planes that almost collide. My takeaway is that patients have to be the safety on their healthcare team. Until healthcare ensures zero errors you must play a larger role in protecting yourself and your loved ones than anyone would want. This does not absolve the hospital of responsibility for your safety. It's just the reality we live in—sometimes hospitals make mistakes and if you want to stay safe, you will have to watch for these mistakes yourself.

Before I left that day, Dr. James gave me a yellow rubber wristband that read, "First Do No Harm," an unofficial part of the Hippocratic Oath that defines a doctor's duty to his or her patients. On my wrist, the band has lived as a constant reminder of the absolute necessity to chip away at James' number of 400,000 medical errors per year until that number is zero. Even one death from medical error is too many.

Until hospitals have zero errors here are hints to help you stay safe in some of the most dangerous hospital situations.

## Minimize your Exposure to Risk

The more minutes an NFL player is in the game, the higher the chance of injury. The same is true in hospitals—the longer your stay, the higher your chance of medical error. In fact, some hospitals have started incentivizing doctors to reduce your stay in the hospital, not just because a shorter stay costs less, but because every hour you stay in the hospital puts you more at risk. It's pretty simple: If your condition permits you to be somewhere other than the hospital, be somewhere other than the hospital. This is definitely something you should bring up with your doctor. You should all be asking, "Does this care need to be done in the hospital or could it be done safely in another setting?" The best hospital experience is one that doesn't happen in the first place.

## Injured on Kickoff

When the NFL found that players were routinely injured on kickoffs, the League responded by moving the kick forward to the 35-yard line so more kicks went unreturned. Now the NFL is considering more changes to make kickoffs even safer. Your entrance to the hospital is your healthcare kickoff and it can be just as dangerous (one of the most dangerous kinds of "transitions," as we'll see elsewhere in this book).

Chances are you enter the hospital through the ER and, unlike your PCP who hopefully has known you for years, you will be a stranger to the ER team. This means that it will be your job to begin to fill the gap of knowledge between your PCP and ER doctor. One good way to do this is to have access to all your important health data. If you have access to a patient portal you can just pull it up on your phone. If you have it in a computer file or other electronic format you can provide it easily as well. If you don't have it electronically then there is nothing wrong with arriving at the ER with a good, old, paper cheat sheet. If all else fails, throw all your medications in a brown paper bag and bring them with you. If you're admitted to the hospital from the ER, your team will need to know not only what you're taking, but how much and when. And if you end up in observation status rather than being admitted, you can always take you own mediation to save money.

In addition to your data, what you say counts. Be sure to share all your signs and symptoms. Don't hold back—every little detail may be important. Usually if you're in the ER, you're in some kind of distress and so it can be good to have your family or another caregiver with you to help fill in any details you forget. Have your family or caregivers there to help fill in these details. Above all else, remember that more is better. More information and more communication will help you enter the hospital safely.

## Tired or Burned out Healthcare Providers

In 2013 the Chargers had the ball on the Redskins' one-yard line, trailing 24-21 with 0:21 on the game clock. Coach Mike McCoy called a run up the middle and when that didn't work, had his quarterback, Philip Rivers, throw the ball twice…incomplete. The Chargers ended up settling for a field goal and then went on to lose in overtime. McCoy was pilloried on sports radio and across the internet for bad play calling. NFL coaches take game preparation to the extreme and later McCoy admitted that he had gone completely overboard, sleeping only a few hours a night during the week before the game. In other words, he was burned out—McCoy lost the game because he had worked too hard.

How many hours has your doctor been awake? How many patients does he or she have to see today? How many patients does your nurse have to take care of today? The answers to these questions may affect your healthcare, so you have the right to know them.

And the answers may surprise you. A recent survey found that 25 percent of hospitalists felt that multiple times in a month, the number of patients they saw in a day exceeded a safe number. Twenty-two percent said that they have ordered costly or unnecessary tests or consults because they didn't have adequate time to properly assess their patients. Likewise, a California study found that nurse-to-patient ratios can affect how many patients die in the hospital. When the nurses they studied had fewer patients, mortality rates improved going from seven to two percent.

There have been days in my career when I have had more patients to see than I felt comfortable with. All doctors have experienced this. Sometimes it's of our own doing, and other times it's out of our control. Sometimes it just happens that a lot of people get sick and come to the hospital on the same night.

Physician burnout is and will continue to be a huge problem for our healthcare system. Physician shortages are a certainty: We are adding more patients, but we still have the same number of doctors, or perhaps fewer than we used to have.

So what can you do if you're faced with an overwhelmed, overworked doctor? First, like anything else, simply being aware can help. If your hospitalist's first visit to see you comes very late in the day or at night, that can hint at a problem. If your doctor seems to be spending very little time in your room, or if you suspect that he or she is seeing a large number of patients, you may want to talk to a patient representative. The same goes for your nurse: if he or she seems too busy or is not responding to your needs, it is fully within your rights to talk with the patient representative or the head nurse.

Don't be afraid to call a time-out. You don't have to confront the doctor or nurse, but letting the hospital know of your concerns may help shed light on the issue. The hospital may look at the doctor's number of patients and the times that he or she sees them each day, and may conclude that your doctor has an excessive burden. In extreme cases, you can always request that another doctor take over your case. The hospital should facilitate this process so that you don't have to confront the doctor.

## Sticky Hands

Lester Hayes played for the Oakland Raiders (my favorite team when I was growing up) and was one of the most-feared cornerbacks in the history of the NFL. He was known for using a sticky substance called Stickum™ on his hands, which in theory helped you catch or hold onto the ball. Much to the dismay of many other players, even some on his own team, he would lather his hands, pads, and even his uniform in the gooey slime. In 1981, the NFL banned Stickum and other sticky substances for good.

Our healthcare system has its own "sticky hands" problem. Studies estimate about one hundred thousand patients die each year from infections acquired in the hospital, making it one of the leading causes of healthcare-related preventable deaths. One out of twenty hospital patients develops a healthcare-acquired infection (HAI). Sadly, many of these infections are caused by bacteria from healthcare workers who have not properly washed their hands. We need to ban sticky hands in hospitals!

In fact, I recently visited a hospital that was on the verge of being closed by the Joint Commission due to poor hand washing and poor monitoring of the problem. This hospital has since corrected the problem, in part by sending "secret shoppers" to watch if doctors and nurses wash their hands. Now technology actually exists to monitor this with a chip. When the hospital room door is opened, the hand cleanser dispenser must be activated, with a chip tracking when this does not occur.

The very best way for healthcare workers to prevent these infections is to wash their sticky hands. Good hand washing would go a long way toward preventing needless deaths. Don't be afraid to ask your doctor, nurse, and any other person who comes into your room to wash their hands. Sanitizing, alcohol-based hand gels are very popular these days and used properly kill some but not all bacteria and viruses. Still, gels are no substitute for washing! And if anyone is going to touch a wound you have or draw your blood, that person should be wearing gloves.

## Foreign Bodies

When in doubt, get it out! That's because any foreign body inside you presents a risk for infection. There are 560,000 catheter-associated urinary tract infections and

250,000 venous catheter infections per year. If you can urinate without needing a tube in your bladder for any reason, it's best not to have one. If you don't need a tube in your vein or artery, you are always better off having it removed as soon as possible.

## The Danger of Immobility

Derrick Thomas was the fourth overall draft pick of the Kansas City Chiefs in 1989 and played his entire stellar career with the team. On January 23, 2000, he was involved in a devastating car accident and was paralyzed from the chest down. While being treated at a Miami hospital he suddenly felt ill and went into cardiopulmonary arrest. He died of a massive blood clot to his lungs. When we lay in hospital beds we can be at risk to develop clots like this in our legs that can travel to our lungs. Hospitals should have a prevention strategy for every patient which can involve air inflated pressure devices or blood thinning shots or pills. You can do your part by getting up and moving (with the right support) when you are cleared to do so.

Like an NFL running back who never stops moving, the sooner and more you get up and move, especially after surgery, the better. Gone are the days when we thought bed rest was best. When it is safe, get moving in order to prevent blood clots and weakness. One study famously took highly trained athletes and put them on bed rest and you would not believe how weak they were at the end of 30 days.

Being immobilized can also put you at risk for bedsores and pressure ulcers. Left untreated, these can go so deep that they can infect your bones. Your nurse should be aware of these protocols and may even call in a nurse who specializes in treating wounds to help prevent these kinds of infections.

## Hitting the Turf

As many as 20 percent of patients fall at least once during their hospital stay. Did you know that when elderly patients fall, it causes death 25 percent of the time? This is just inside the hospital. Outside the hospital, as many as one-third of elderly patients fall over the course of a year. Falls are the number one cause of injury in this older age group. As more and more baby boomers enter their senior years, this epidemic of falls is sure to grow.

Hospitals try to reduce the risk of falls with bed alarms that blare an alert when patients try to get out of bed, bed rails, labeling the patient as a fall risk, beds that are very low to the ground and, like the NFL, helmets. I've seen fall risk patients decorate their helmets!

If you or a loved one is in the hospital, your best strategy is simply to be aware of the risk of falls. When in doubt, it's best to have a family member stay in the hospital to make sure your loved one doesn't get up without the appropriate supervision. Many patients, particularly seniors, can get confused in the hospital, making them prone to ignoring fall precautions. When my father fell and broke his hip outside the hospital, we took turns staying in the hospital after his surgery to make sure he was thinking clearly enough not to get up on his own. It may sound like overkill, but until you are confident that your loved one will not try to get up without help, this is the safest way to try and prevent serious complications.

## Medications: Offensive Weapons or Bad Chemistry

Medications are one of the greatest weapons we have to defeat disease but they also can do a lot of harm. Adverse drug events are defined by the Agency for Healthcare Research and Quality (AHRQ) as "Harm experienced by a patient as a result of exposure to medication." They account for about 700,000 ER visits and 100,000 hospitalizations a year. They happen to 5 percent of hospitalized patients, making adverse drug events the most common medical error.

Keep yourself safe by making sure that you and the healthcare team have your heads in the game at medication time. You should be told the name of every medication you are given and why you are taking it. Before you are started on any medication, the risks and benefits should be discussed, including all side effects. Your current medications should always be taken into consideration to avoid dangerous inter-actions. You should get all your medications on time and just as it can be dangerous to take medicines that are prescribed poorly, it can be dangerous *not* to take some critical medicines like blood thinners, seizure medications, antibiotics, or immu-nosuppressants. According to the AHRQ one-third of adults take 5 or more medications. I see patients taking more than 20 at times! This is called poly-pharmacy, and the risk of adverse events and interactions is enormous with this many medica-tions. Always ask, "Why am I on this and do I need it?"

## Delay of Game

"I was admitted to the hospital last night at 11:30 p.m. Now it's 5:00 pm the next day and I still haven't seen a doctor!" Unfor-tunately, this may sound all too familiar. While in the hospital, regulations dictate that you see a doctor every twenty-four hours. That may seem like a bare minimum, but believe me, sometimes patients go for days without seeing a doctor. This can be due to poor scheduling or to errors like computer snafus or the ball being dropped in the handoff between one doctor and the next.

Delay of game is important because delays in your care increase the risk of misdiagnosis and delayed diagnosis. If you feel like it takes an unusually long time to see a doctor, it's very important that you notify your nurse. If your nurse cannot get a doctor to come and see you, then ask to talk to the hospital's patient representative.

## Eye in the Sky

The NFL now has a trainer up in the press box to watch every play. The league calls this their "eye in the sky." It came about after Redskins quarterback Colt McCoy was injured without sideline personnel or coaches seeing how. When I spoke with NFL Head and Spine Committee member, Dr. Margot Putukian, director of Athletic Medicine at Princeton, she told me that after the injury, NFL physicians and trainers immediately held a meeting. They could not believe that fans at home were able to watch the Colt McCoy play five times from many angles and yet the coaches and trainers were only able to see what their eyes had shown them in real-time. It wasn't long after that the NFL instituted this "eye in the sky." In the hospital, an eye in the sky can keep you safe too. Your agent or family can be that eye in the sky for you.

In football and in healthcare, the eye in the sky can be technological too. Kevin M. Guskiewicz is a nationally recognized expert on sports concussions and, recently, the dean of the School of Arts and Sciences at my old training program, UNC–Chapel Hill. When I visited the program, Guskiewicz and Dr. Mario Ciocca, head of the university's sports medicine program, showed me around and I was amazed at several things—the loud music the coach allowed during practice, the accelerometers inside helmets to measure the force of impacts, and the computer able to track every hit in real-time. If a hit went over the allowable force the system alerted a coach who would check the player. Healthcare is starting to use electronic triggers as well, for example electronic medical records that can alert medical teams to possible drug interactions or questionable dosages.

To end on a more positive note, healthcare is aware of high levels of danger and errors in hospitals and aggressive, proactive steps have started to reduce this danger. When I spoke with Patrick Conway, he shared that for the first time in history harm decreased in hospitals, citing a 9 percent reduction in infections during the years 2010–2012, resulting in approximately 520,000 fewer infections and 15,000 saved lives. Even more recent data from the ARHQ showed a 17 percent reduction in harm from "hospital acquired conditions" from 2010–2014, saving 87,000 lives.

Progress is being made and credit should be given, but we still have a long way to go to zero. Don't fear hospitals, but don't get lulled into a "safety bubble" in which you expect the system to be solely responsible for your wellbeing.

# CHAPTER 17:
## Fumbling the Handoff
## Healthcare's #1 Safety Problem

By now you've heard me describe healthcare as composed of "teams of teams." Nowhere is this more true than in the hospital. First there's the hospital team composed of everyone who works there. Then that team is divided into smaller teams for each floor or unit. The operating room and departments like radiology and pathology are other teams. The social workers and case managers are on teams as well. Some doctors that are employed by the hospital similarly work with and across these teams. Next level away are doctors and teams that don't work directly for the hospital but have contracted to provide one specific kind of care, for example ER services or hospitalist or anesthesia. They live in a world between the team that is their own company and the hospital team.

Finally, there are doctors and others that come to the hospital but have no business relationship at all. Some private practice doctors come to visit their patients in the hospital but that is it. Home health companies and hospices and skilled nursing facilities and rehab centers send their representatives there to get referrals. Sometimes there are case managers that work for insurance companies that will make rounds in the hospital. Some doctors might be hired by insurance companies to oversee the care of patients who have a certain insurance.

Within, among and between all of these teams, there are handoffs. You are the ball. You can go from the ER to the ICU or a hospital room, from one room to another, or from the hospital to home, a skilled nursing facility, a rehabilitation hospital, or even to another hospital. Each one of these handoffs is another opportunity for healthcare to drop the ball.

Think about an NFL handoff. When a quarterback takes the snap and then hands off to the running back, there's a split second in which both players have the ball. Healthcare requires the same mechanics—when any team or team member hands a patient to anyone (or anywhere) else, it takes a coordinated transfer of information and responsibility. Otherwise you can end up like NFL fumble leader Brett Favre, or, more precisely, like the ball he so often dropped onto the frozen tundra of Lambeau Field. Here are some of the most important and most dangerous hospital handoff situations and, most importantly, how to stay safe.

## ER to Hospital

If you are admitted to the hospital from the ER, a very important handoff occurs—either to your PCP if he or she works at the hospital and will be managing your care, or to a hospitalist who will act as your interim head coach while you're admitted. Keep in mind that even if your PCP is able to manage your hospital care, you might be better off transferring to a hospitalist who has more experience and expertise in managing patients in the hospital setting. I call this a dilemma of *continuity* vs. *capability*. If you have many complex medical problems and your PCP has the skills to take care of you in a hospital setting, sticking with the continuity of someone who knows you and your health history is probably best. If your PCP doesn't go to the hospital often and has not taken care of complex, hospitalized patients on a regular basis you should consider temporarily replacing your head coach with the interim head coach of a hospitalist. This decision is best discussed when you have your first visit with your PCP and not at the time of an emergency. Ask if your PCP still takes care of patients in the hospital. Ask how often your PCP sees hospitalized patients. Ask if your PCP has a preferred hospitalist or hospitalist group to manage your care if you are admitted. It may be an uncomfortable conversation, but if you believe your care is best managed by a hospitalist and not your PCP, you can ask your ER doctor for this change and it must be honored. Consider asking the ER doctor or the staff which hospitalist they would recommend.

ER doctors really want to do a few things: Stabilize you, determine if you have to stay or can go home, rule out very bad things, make a diagnosis, and treat you if possible. When they are close to finishing these important tasks, they will reach out to your PCP to get further information and to do a handoff. If you are able to go home from the ER this call brings your PCP into the game plan. However, you may still need to pick up the ball if there is a fumble, for example if a test is pending when you leave. Despite the handoff your PCP may forget that you had a urine culture but you can close that gap and remind them on your follow up visit. By leaving with a record of your

ER care in hand you can keep your own accurate record and bring it to your visit.

If you need to be admitted, the ER doctor will have a conversation about your handoff with this person who will be taking over the management of your care—typically by phone but sometimes in person. The nurses will do a handoff to their counterparts up on the hospital wards as well. In the best of all worlds, this is a seamless handoff with no delays, but this is rarely the case. You will sometimes have to wait in the ER for up to 24 hours before a bed on the ward opens up and then wait some more until a hole in the ER doc's schedule lines up with a hole in the PCP or hospitalist's schedule.

This time during which you are officially admitted to the hospital but are physically still in the ER can be a dangerous no-man's land—a gap in the handoff between the quarter-back and running back. The busy ER nurses and doctors have moved on to other cases and although they will still be responsible for you, they can get distracted. And the doctor that will be overseeing your care in the hospital hasn't joined the team yet. Again, if you think the game plan is not being executed, call a timeout. If tests that were to be done don't seem to occur or medications that you need are not given on time, call a timeout.

Another piece of the handoff between an ER doctor and your hospitalist (if not your PCP) is communication with the office that manages your day-to-day care. This communication should help your hospitalist fill in any missing data, better understand your preferences and goals, and can be a valuable way for your hospitalist to get insight into your care that comes from knowing you over time. If this handoff does not occur or is done poorly you will have to pick up the ball.

This is another very common point in the healthcare handoff where hospitals drop the ball. Ask your hospital team if they've spoken with your PCP's office. If not, you may have to contact your PCP's office to let them know you are in the hospital and to request that copies of your medical record or other important information be emailed or faxed to the hospital. In this communication, you may also need your PCP to send information to your insurance company.

Need another quick peek at the playbook? Here you go: When you enter a hospital through the ER, make sure the ER doctor hands off to a hospitalist. Make sure your hospitalist contacts your PCP's office. And if you feel like your care is being fumbled, call a timeout!

## Ward to Ward

You have a bed. You have a room. You're all settled into whatever movie you've chosen on the room's entertainment system. And then it's time to pack up and move. This typically occurs when moving from a more intense setting like the intensive care unit to a less intense area, like a step-down unit. Sometimes if you have surgery you will go to a different floor for recovery before transitioning to a longer-term room. Room changes can also happen due to the realities of reshuffling. For example, if a patient has a high infection risk he or she might need a private room and you might need to be moved to another space.

No matter why you move, when you move to another room your doctors will usually stay the same but your nurses will not. (In a new successful model of care, doctors are assigned to a specific unit and so if you move, your hospitalist would change as well—you can ask about this.) The big handoff in switching rooms is between nurses and the most common fumble is in medications. Even though medications should be documented in your chart sometimes there is misunderstanding about whether and when a medication was given. It's a terrible truth that sometimes patients have to recover the fumble of a hospital handoff—it's not fair, it's not right, and it's not safe. But despite all that, sometimes it's the harsh reality of current hospitals. If you switch rooms, check in with your new nursing team about your medications. Just this reminder can help them take another, closer look at your game plan and make sure they're not dropping the ball.

## Team to Team

When my children were little I used to read them a book called *Are You My Mother?* in which a baby bird asks different animals if they are his mother. The hospital can feel the same way— patients continually ask, "Are you my doctor?" Who are all these people in white coats visiting your room? Which one of them is actually managing your care?

One reason you see so many new faces is that your PCP or hospitalist doesn't work 24/7 and may hand off your care to a partner or colleague for portions of your stay. Also, some PCPs take turns covering all of a practice's patients who happen to be in the hospital, and if it's not your PCP's turn while you are admitted, you may receive care from a partner. Hospitalist-to-hospitalist handoffs are even more common. Most hospitalists work in shifts with the most common rotation being seven days on and seven days off. The average hospital stay is about 4.5 days so you may have the same hospitalist the entire time but more often you will have at least two and maybe more. When there's a trade, expect that your new doctor will need to ask questions that seem redundant—haven't you already gone over this? Yes, but with a different doctor. Your outgoing hospitalist should let you know he or she will be handing your care off and who your new doctor will be. Ideally, the outgoing hospitalist will be available to answer any questions should they arise by phone in those first days with your new hospitalist.

In addition to these "regular" doctor handoffs, there's a special kind of handoff that happens if you are admitted at night. In that case, an overnight hospitalist will take your "history and physical" and then hand off care to another hospitalist in the morning. Really, an overnight hospitalist can be kind of like a placeholder for the doctor who takes over when the sun comes up. This is an important handoff! It means that your entire history and physical was taken by a person who will never actually manage your care. Treat this situation just like the handoff between the ER and the hospital. All of your info is going to someone new and it's worth keeping a close eye on the ball to make sure nothing gets dropped.

## The Biggest Handoff: Going Home

Leaving the hospital for home or even for another facility like a rehabilitation hospital or skilled nursing facility is the most dangerous and risky transition of all. We called your admission to the hospital a "kickoff" but, really, the game begins when you leave.

Counterintuitively, your discharge game plan should start the second you enter the hospital. From the time you are admitted, start to think, "When will I be safe to go home and what will I need in order to go home safely and stay there?" Checking off these critical criteria should be a major goal while in the hospital. Then make sure you work with your doctor to write and share your discharge game plan. This is a hugely important step in your ability to run with the ball once you leave the hospital. Your doctor probably has a pretty clear picture of what is possible for you in the hospital, but you're the one who knows what it's like to be home. You know what you can do, and you can be realistic about what you *will* do, once you leave the support and care of the hospital. Make sure you understand your discharge plan and feel like the instructions are feasible.

NFL coaches should know their players' capabilities but ultimately it is the players themselves that know themselves best. If your game plan involves something that you will not be able to do, whatever it is, call a timeout. It could involve cost or a medication or the ability to get to an appointment. Remember, the hospital is practice—don't wait until you are in the heat of the game to be realistic about parts of the game plan that were never really going to work for you.

Here are two things that make patients leave with an unrealistic game plan: First, a patient wants to please the doctor or just get out of the hospital and so agrees with the discharge plan without really accepting the challenge of its instructions; or second, a patient doesn't really listen to the discharge plan, figuring that he or she can nod their way through the instructions and then return to business as usual once he or she gets home. Your discharge plan is an opportunity. It's an opportunity to make the changes that can help you not only go home but *stay* home. Accepting this all-important handoff can be one of the most powerful things you do for your health.

Try a technique we call "teach back." Once your doctor talks you through a part of your discharge plan, pretend as if you are teaching the doctor this section. Don't just repeat it back or read it from the page; teach your doctor what to "do" at home. If your doctor sees a misunderstanding in your teaching, you can work together to ensure your understanding. Make sure you understand your diagnosis and any question marks that still exist. Make sure you know what procedures were performed and what your recovery or limitations after these procedures will be. Make sure you understand what tests have been performed and any others that are still pending or are likely options for the future. Of course, make absolutely sure you understand your medicines—what are you taking, when, how much, and what is each medicine supposed to do for you? Some patients are on so many medications just because doctors keep adding them without taking a hard look at reducing others. This is not good for you financially or medically unless each new medication is absolutely necessary. Leaving the hospital is a good time to re-evaluate your medications.

Like an NFL quarterback who runs the option, some of the plays you take home from the hospital will be set in stone, but others will be, "if this, then that." For example, if your dressing falls off this is how to change it; or if your blood sugar is this number take this amount of insulin; or if these symptoms develop this is when you should seek further care. Doctors call this last step a "notify when…" Maybe if you notice redness or drainage after wound care, you should check in with your PCP. With these "notify whens" make sure you not only know when you should seek care, but how to go about doing it. Write the phone numbers you should call or the addresses of the places you should go in your discharge plan.

And this brings us to another essential piece of your discharge game plan: *Write this all down!* There is no way you can remember everything you are supposed to do at home. You should work with your doctor to understand your discharge game plan, but realize that you don't have to memorize it. Use your plan as a cheat sheet. Your goal is to make sure *everything* is on that cheat sheet. Later you'll want to use this as your version of the NFL's video instant replay. Did the nose of the ball *really* reach the goal line? What does that reception look like from 15 different angles? Your cheat sheet lets you go back to the tape to review and reinterpret that conversation you had with your doctor about your discharge instructions.

In fact, I recently spoke with Dr. David Langer, chairman of the Department of Neurosurgery at Lenox Hill Hospital in New York City, who mentioned that he has started videotaping discharge instructions. The NFL uses film to review performance—why shouldn't healthcare? When I brought up my football analogy with Dr. Langer, he said that his team had already started thinking about these discharge videos as "highlight reels." He is studying the results of these videos now, which can include walk-through of patient's scans and test results.

In addition to leaving the hospital with your game plan in hand, be it paper or multimedia, back up this plan with copies of all your medical records. More and more hospitals are allowing patients full access to their medical records—either paper or electronic. The more you can get, the better. Make sure your records include not only the test results that came back while you were in the hospital, but information about any tests that were ordered with the results still pending. After discharge, you will be following up with your PCP and if he or she doesn't know about these tests, how will your PCP know to check on them?

Know your discharge game plan. Make it a realistic play-book that can guide your actions at home. And use your medical records to close the information gap with your PCP. When you go home you are not only the all-important ball, but you are the running back who carries it. At home, you are responsible for protecting yourself. Use the hospital to learn how to keep yourself safe and healthy once the real kickoff happens and you head out through those hospital doors.

## General Rules for Ball Protection in the Hospital

Don't forget that the biggest handoff is when you *leave* the hospital for home or for a rehab or skilled nursing facility! That's why we have a whole chapter on that later. In the meantime, now that we've looked at some specific handoff situations, let's dial in some general rules for hospital hand-offs. No matter where you're transferred to or what new person shows up in your room, use these rules to make sure your handoff is safe:

### THE WORST HANDOFFS ARE NONE AT ALL

Your doctors and nurses should let you know when a handoff is happening and who your new provider will be. It's fine to ask your doctor for this information. Just say, "When you place my care in another doctor's hands, please let me know so that I can be an informed part of the team."

### ASK ABOUT THE HANDOFF

Since handoffs are a particularly dangerous time for patients, good doctors don't mind you asking how they will be handled.

For example, you might say, "How will your partner know that I am to be discharged in the morning?" Your doctor should say something like, "I'll make sure to tell her all about your case before she takes over."

## IF YOU THINK THERE HAS BEEN A BAD HANDOFF, CALL A TIMEOUT

If a new doctor, nurse, or any team member comes into your room and seems to be talking about a different patient or doesn't seem to understand all the key elements of your case, don't be afraid to call a timeout! Ask your team member to make sure they're looking at the right chart and that they know the important aspects of your care.

## BE PREPARED TO PICK UP THE BALL

In the event of a bad handoff, you might have to recover the fumble. This is one reason it's so important for you to keep track of your healthcare information during your stay in the hospital. That information can be as important to your health as the most powerful medicine. If it looks like the ball has come loose, you can be the one who picks it up and recovers the fumble by providing your team with the information it needs.

## IF THERE ARE TOO MANY HANDOFFS

If you see too many hospitalists or head coaches during your stay, call a timeout. Remember your hospitalist is the head coach guiding the big picture of your care, coordinating it with all your other coaches or specialists. Your hospitalist writes all the key orders. If you have had more than three during your stay, call a timeout and ask if you can stick with one for the rest of your stay. The longer you stay the less this may be possible, but it never hurts to ask.

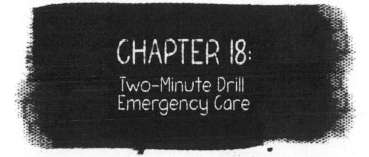

# CHAPTER 18:
## Two-Minute Drill
## Emergency Care

Growing up in postwar Philadelphia, there was a blond boy who never missed a game of street football or "backyard brawl," a game in which one brave kid picked up the ball and bolted for his life as a swarm of neighborhood kids attempted to maul the lone victim. With five siblings and a voracious teenage boy appetite, he learned early to devour anything resembling food when it hit the table. So why was he losing weight? And lately it seemed like he was the only one in his bedroom crowded with brothers and sisters that had to get up in the middle of the night to pee. He drank glasses and glasses of water but was thirsty all the time. Kids were starting to snicker as he asked his teacher for yet another restroom pass.

Finally, his mom scheduled a doctor's visit. He didn't really know why he had never liked doctors—probably the shots. After the exam and without a hint of indecision, the doctor brusquely offered his diagnosis: there was nothing wrong with the boy. The boy and the mother didn't speak on the way home. Despite the doctor's assurances, they both knew something was wrong.

After six more weeks of weight loss, drinking and peeing something went very wrong. At first the boy thought he was having a bad dream. He was taking deeper and deeper breaths, but seemed to get less and less air. Shaking it off, he tried to sit up in bed but his arms and legs were lifeless and wouldn't follow his commands. Everything had the hazy, cold, muffled feel of being trapped under a frozen lake. He screamed with his last ounce of strength and his mother rushed in. She knew this was it. The boy was dying.

His dad raced in, grabbed him in his quilt, and tossed the boy into the back seat of the car. Running traffic lights they sped to Bryn Mawr Hospital as the boy's breathing got faster and faster, racing like the car. When the car stopped at the emergency room, his mom jumped out with the boy and sprinted past security into the waiting area. Nurses instinctually grabbed the child, his eyes rolling back in his head as they hurried him onto a stretcher. His lips were blue, his tiny frame gray, contorted with each desperate attempt for more air. A team of doctors, nurses, and orderlies descended on the room as his heart beat faded, slower and slower on the monitor. His parents were rushed out of the fray.

Then a confident young doctor strode into the room, smelled fruit on the boy's breath and immediately ordered insulin. Remarkably the boy began to awaken from his coma. How could their family doctor have missed a classic case of diabetes? When he was moved to a regular room, the boy asked if he could watch TV. That night of December 28, 1958, that

13-year-old boy watched the "Greatest Game" in NFL history. That boy was my dad.

An emergency room is like a good backup quarterback: You never want to use it but when you need it, you're glad it's there. You twist your knee in a weekend football game or slice your finger open at work. You develop chest pain and trouble breathing or you suddenly lose the ability to talk. You need a flu shot or you think your child has an ear infection but you have to work. Where do you turn?

To begin with, think like an NFL fan looking for tickets to a game. Going to the ER is like buying tickets from a scalper standing outside the stadium—you don't need an appointment and can go at the last minute but it is also the most expensive. And using your regular healthcare team, there are so many unknowns. When will you be seen? Which doctor will you see? Like paying for tickets at the last minute, everything is more expensive in an ER—every pill and shot and procedure. Just as a scalper has to make back the money they paid for the tickets, hospitals have to charge high ER rates to pay for all that equipment and all those experts ready not just for your emergency but for anything, any time.

But the ER is only one of many options for acute care. In the modern game of medicine, you have many choices—an ER attached to a hospital, a freestanding ER, an urgent care in or out of a hospital, a retail clinic, a work-affiliated clinic, your PCP, or even a virtual visit with or without video. This chapter is about which option to use, when to use it, and how to get the most value once you're there.

## You Can't Predict an Emergency

As a kid, my favorite television show was Emergency about two paramedics in Los Angeles. We used to play our own version of the show, making my little sister act the part of the car accident victim. And who can forget the show ER, which launched George Clooney's career? Now thanks to the wonder of cable TV, you can have a firsthand view of real ERs along with Emmy shoe-ins like "Sex Brought Me to the ER" and "Untold Stories of the ER."

TV dramas love the ER for obvious reasons: late nights, alcohol, drugs, guns, violence, and a neverending conveyor belt of critical life-and-death decisions. The very first rotation of my medical internship was in the ER and it was one of the scariest times in my life as a doctor. It's a place where ordering Tylenol can escalate in minutes to shocking a person back to life. You see things in the ER that are hard to believe. Like a woman who came in one evening, vomiting and obviously pregnant. Only, she wasn't. It turned out to be a case of pseudocyesis, a condition of false pregnancy in which a woman believes so strongly she is pregnant that it can cause physical symptoms. Until we had triple-checked the test results, she had me fooled—baby bump and all (and with five children, I should know!). Then there was the time on the overnight shift the radio blared with the news, "incoming multiple GSW to the head, young female victim, out for early am run!" GSW stands for "gunshot wound" and I knew that my former wife sometimes took early morning walks in that neighborhood. When the patient arrived, it wasn't my wife. The female gunshot victim died in the OR, age 26, and I still worried that my wife might be out walking with the killer on the loose.

There's a superstition in the ER against using the "Q" word: quiet. As soon as someone says it's quiet, all hell breaks loose. I remember one night an intern yawned and remarked on how quiet it had been...right before a female bodybuilder on PCP was wheeled in with three orderlies holding her down. She proceeded to toss two of the large men off her chest and then took on the ER's security staff. I joined the fray with several doctors and nurses and finally one lucky nurse hit her thigh with a sedative and the bodybuilder went down. A couple days later, I started lifting weights at the gym again—a practice I had given up during med school.

Then there was the time I was in training and was called in to help the ER doc with a case. All I saw was the chart hanging on the patient's door. It was Florida and the man had been bit by a coral snake. Of course, in cases of animal bite, it's always good to bring the animal with you if you can so that doctors can make the most informed diagnosis. But if it's poisonous, please don't bring it in alive! His chart informed his providers that he had, in fact, brought the coral snake with him. I remember insisting that we kill or remove the snake before I would see the patient.

Even if you know that you have a dangerous health condition, you probably won't be able to predict when you will need acute care. Then there are those completely unexpected emergencies—the broken leg or bee sting that closes your throat despite many previous uneventful stings. Here is how to manage these times when you need care and you need it fast.

## DON'T HESITATE WHEN EVERY MINUTE COUNTS

You will never be able to take back those minutes you wait to call 911. Studies have proven that quick action with a heart attack not only saves lives that day, but keeps heart tissue from dying. Similarly, the clot busting medication given for new strokes has a critical 12-hour window with every hour saving some brain tissue. There's no way to make a complete list of all the symptoms or accidents that require emergency care, but if you cannot breathe or your heart rate is too high or low, or you find yourself with unexplained neurological symptoms like confusion or inability to speak, err on the side of caution and call 911.

College football players talk about the realization in their first NFL practice or game that the "speed is on another level." That's the ER. In this book, we've defined "value" in healthcare as the relationship of quality to cost, but in the case of the ER "quality" can be less a spectrum than the black-or-white difference between whether you live or die. What is the "quality" of saving your life? I would say that in emergency care, this life-saving quality is infinitely important, which makes the cost irrelevant. In emergencies, the risk of a bad outcome is so great that the most expensive option—the emergency room or even calling 911 to be taken to the emergency room—is the best value always.

Be aware that in most cases ambulance services will be obligated to take you to the closest ER, maybe at a hospital that is out of your insurance network, and if it turns out you don't truly have an emergency condition, you may also have to pay for the ambulance ride. Still, I would argue not to worry about these details in such a fearful and frantic setting. Save your life now and fight the bill later (using the resources in section III). But avoid using an ambulance as a medical Uber—if you clearly don't need one, it's likely to be the most expensive cab ride of your life.

Given the importance of immediate care for heart attacks and strokes, I include more information specific to these topics below. Please take this very seriously. I cannot tell you how many times a patient has told me, "Well I woke up and couldn't feel my arm. I thought I slept on it wrong but the feeling would not come back, and then I had trouble seeing or talking, but I thought it would just go away and I tried to go back to sleep." In these critical minutes, precious brain or heart tissue may be dying.

## IF YOU THINK YOU ARE HAVING A HEART ATTACK

You may hear a doctor refer to heart attack as an acute myocardial infarction or acute M.I. The signs of an MI may include chest pain (squeezing, like someone sitting on your chest, or discomfort of any kind), shortness of breath, nausea, vomiting, pain in the jaw, or pain radiating down either arm. Women may have more atypical symptoms with more jaw or back pain. If you think you are having a heart attack call 911; do not drive. Most important, getting to an ER in the fastest way possible can save heart damage and possibly your life. Hospitals are measured on what is called door-to-balloon time or the time from when you roll through the ER door until you get a special procedure using a catheter with a small balloon that opens blocked arteries to our heart. In studies, every second of this door-to-balloon time makes a difference and that statistic measured in a ticking stopwatch doesn't even take into account the possible delay of discounting your symptoms or putting off getting care.

## IF YOU THINK YOU ARE HAVING A STROKE

The signs of a stroke include numbness, weakness, difficulty speaking or understanding speech, confusion, changes in your vision or facial expression including drooping, passing out or losing consciousness, or any sudden neurologic symptom. The American Stroke Association uses the acronym F.A.S.T. to make it easy to remember when you should call 911—F: Face drooping; A: Arm weakness; S: Speech difficulty; T: Time to call 911. Take it seriously. In a stroke, blood clots prevent your brain from getting the oxygen it needs and every minute without oxygen more brain tissue dies. An ER's stroke care critical team can also treat your brain with protective and nourishing medicines that can stop new damage and even reverse some of the damage associated with a stroke. Getting this treatment soon enough can be the difference between regaining brain function and losing it forever.

## When You Can Choose Your ER

I remember working at an ER one Sunday afternoon when a car sped up, tossed a 14-year-old onto the curb, and drove off. The boy was covered in blood, having been shot multiple times in the head in a gang-related incident. We rushed the kid into the operating room but it was too late. If he had had critical care in an ambulance on his way to the hospital, he might have lived. This illustrates an important point: When you need care right away, calling an ambulance is the quickest way to get it.

Then there are times when an emergency isn't quite so critical and you can have a friend or family member drive you to the ER. Now you have some choices. Generally, there are three kinds of emergency rooms, those embedded in a hospital, free-standing ER's affiliated with a hospital, and standalone ER's that have no hospital affiliation. You may have noticed free-standing ER's popping up all over your neighborhood. Don't confuse them with urgent care centers. Urgent care centers typically have family practice or internal medicine doctors who are not board certified in emergency medicine. Even ER's not within a hospital have the same physicians and most of the diagnostic and treatment equipment you would expect to find in a hospital ER, particularly the equipment needed to treat common emergencies. However, the goal of most of these standalone centers is to stabilize you, evaluate your needs, and then, depending on your condition, send you home or transfer you to a regular hospital.

If you have a relationship with a hospital and can choose which ER you visit, it's a no-brainer to have your friend or family member take you to the ER attached to that hospital. This is especially true if it is likely you will need to stay in the hospital. For example, if you have chronic lung disease and know the symptoms of exacerbation, you might know that from the ER you will be spending a couple days in a bed. Of course, you should go to the ER that feeds into the hospital you know. The same is true if you're having a baby or complications from pregnancy: Go through the ER in the hospital that you know (unless it's too far away).

Even if you don't have a favorite hospital, there are times when it's best to go to a hospital ER. For example, if you have a broken bone or other injuries that will require surgery, there's no reason to go to a freestanding ER—you're just going to be transferred to a hospital for surgery anyway. Why waste time and money, and risk a more involved handoff by moving between systems?

One big difference between freestanding ERs that are and aren't affiliated with hospitals is that hospital-associated ERs are inspected and regulated by the Joint Commission, the same body that regulates hospitals themselves. Also, these hospital-affiliated ERs are required to accept Medicaid and Medicare. Freestanding ERs not associated with hospitals are owned by private companies and are unlikely to take Medicare and Medicaid.

Let's look at value in these settings. First, due to the potential for error or infection, the ER itself is dangerous and so if you don't really need acute care, the best "value" is to stay out of the ER entirely. On the other hand, if you need immediate stabilization, quality is life and death and cost is not an issue—the best "value" is the ER that is closest. On the other hand, for issues that will be handled as an outpatient completely within the ER, quality depends only on the ER and most will work just fine—the best "value" is the one that is most convenient and least expensive. Consider seeing which ERs in your area have apps that show their wait times. When your ER need is straightforward, you might as well spend as little time as possible sitting in the lobby.

It's in the middle ground between acute emergencies that require stabilization and low-level ER needs that will be easily handled that complexity comes into play. In these cases, you have the luxury of worrying about both quality and cost. And in almost all situations, you're best going to the ER of the hospital you know. For one thing, if your PCP or a hospitalist who knows you can visit you in the ER, he or she may be able to make the call to send you home when an ER doctor would have to make a more conservative call and admit you. Avoiding a hospital admission is a huge saving in time and money, and if you don't really need to be admitted, it is also a huge saving in the quality of your care (we've already seen how dangerous hospitals can be). Then if you do need to be admitted, you will have access to doctors you already know, again increasing the quality of your care. There's also a better chance your health records will be there waiting for you. Sure, another hospital's ER should be able to request your records from your PCP or home hospital, but if you have the choice, why give healthcare another handoff to fumble the ball?

## ER vs. Urgent Care

Now we're in the thick of it. The choice to go to an expensive and inconvenient ER versus a quick and easy urgent care clinic can be a tough one. In this case, you have to do what we all do in healthcare, namely triage. Triage literally means "separate out" which is appropriate, as the process of medical triage is one of separating out your options. If your only options are to call 911 or do nothing, the choice is usually pretty clear. But between these two and especially on the cusp of ER versus urgent care, the decision isn't nearly so clear. Again, let the idea of *value* be your guide—make it a decision of quality over cost.

The first step of self-triage is separating out the conditions that don't require medical attention at all. These cases are certainly the easiest on the wallet! From apps to websites to calling your doctor's office, there are a lot of decision support tools vying for your eyes. I remember when my son was five months old and I was taking care of him while my former wife worked a 12-hour shift as a nurse. I was a second-year medical student and knew just enough to scare the hell out of myself. My son seemed more sleepy that day but at first I was not concerned. Then when I tried to wake him, he wasn't quite as alert as he usually was. I called my wife and she reassured me—she was a pediatric nurse and knew more than I did. However, as the day wore on I began reading my pediatrics textbook and was convinced my son had a severe infection or sepsis. When my wife got home, we woke him up and very briefly, we thought we saw his eyes roll back in his head. That's it! We rushed to the children's hospital where my wife worked only to have my son wake up completely fine—no fever, normal, smiling with all the nurses taking turns holding him. He cooed and they all laughed. New parents might not be the best at self-triage, especially if one of them is a medical student!

But in general, it's better to make the conservative call when dealing with self-triage. Your process should stop with self-triage only if you can reasonably rule out the possibility that anything is seriously wrong. If you can't, it's time to step up to the next level.

Now is a good time to call your PCP. Start with a call to their nurse, the earlier in the day the better. Even for things that you will eventually end up handling in an urgent care or minute clinic, I prefer starting with your team. They know you, they have your record and they may help you avoid a visit altogether. For example, a urinary tract infection can often be handled over the phone. You can also find out if your PCP's office has the right equipment like X-ray machines or the ability to suture a cut if that is what you need. If they don't the office may triage you to an urgent care clinic that does.

If it is not during business hours, you still might be able to get your questions answered by calling your PCP. Many primary care offices, especially those that are designated patient-centered medical homes (PCMH) or in the new value-care models, are required to have expanded hours and after-hours phone coverage. You might not be able to reach your doctor, but you will get a partner or nurse. And a big advantage of calling your PCP first is that the person on the other end of the phone will have access to your health record, which can help in the triage and medical decision-making process.

If you can't reach your PCP's office or don't get a timely callback, you might see if you have access to a nurse on-call through your work or insurance company. Just as your PCP has access to your health records, an insurance nurse has access to your insurance records and can help add information about in- and out-of-network options for care.

I realize that calling your doctor or insurance company is not the place most of you will start. Most of us start with Dr. Google. That's fine! Google is a great place to learn which signs and symptoms to consider when you actually have these conversations with professionals. But don't rely on Google alone—in addition to scaring yourself into insisting on care you might not need, you may end up missing something very important.

If self-triage and then phone triage concludes that you need to be seen, or you get nowhere and decide you must be seen, then again I suggest at least considering starting with your PCP. Even if your doctor is booked, many offices will work you in with a nurse practitioner or physician's assistant the same day. I was amazed to see the head of the Cleveland Clinic say their goal was to have patients seen the same day if necessary. Remember that continuity of care is a big deal when evaluating quality—whenever possible, go with the team you know and that knows you.

That is, unless it doesn't *matter* if the team knows you. For example, a flu shot is a flu shot no matter where you get it. Might as well go to the most convenient urgent care (or better yet, maybe you can get your flu shot for free through your work!). If you have insurance, the cost of visiting your PCP is likely the same as the cost of visiting an urgent care facility, namely the amount of your co-pay. That said, if you're paying out-of-pocket, urgent care is cheaper.

If you end up going to an urgent care or other facility that is outside your PCP or hospital system, make sure you get a record of your visit and ask them to send a record to your PCP. Closing this gap of care is critical to keeping your team on the same page. Remember, you are working between teams of teams in this case. The urgent care is playing in the NHL and your team is in the NFL. They will not naturally talk or communicate on a regular basis. You have to be the connection. This is a case in which the ball is more likely than not to hit the turf and, unfortunately, it's your job to pick it up.

## Minute and Retail Clinics

Retail medical clinics can be very convenient and less expensive than other options, but there's a reason for that—you may not see a doctor and most retail clinics have very limited tests available. Be aware of the limitations—most won't offer stitches and it's easy to blow past their care ability and end up in an urgent care or ER anyway. If your condition has the potential to be at all complex, you'll want to see a doctor who will be on the lookout for symptoms or combinations of symptoms that can be red flags. That said, these retail clinics are great for very simple treatments like evaluating the use of antibiotics for ear infections or UTIs or for flu shots. The care will also be outside the umbrella of your PCP and you will need to ask that records be sent.

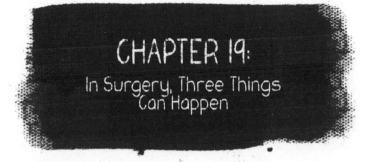

# CHAPTER 19:
## In Surgery, Three Things Can Happen

My mother had a bunion on her big toe. Over time, the big toe started to turn in at an angle, pointing at her other toes. This isn't a completely uncommon ailment. Though the cause is not entirely known, inward-pointing big toes tend to run in families and not only are they more common in women but wearing heels can make it even worse. Over time, my mom got more and more frustrated with the look of her crooked toe, and her new foot shape severely restricted her shoe selection.

Despite these annoyances she was completely pain free. She tried some of the non-surgical treatments like orthotics and roomy shoes but to no avail. Every day she woke up looking at that bunion. Surely she could get it fixed, she concluded. Mind you it had almost no impact functionally on her life at all. Still, she went to see an orthopedic doctor at the preeminent hospital and medical school in town. He was more than eager to offer a surgical solution to her toe, bragging about how straight her new toe would be. Without discussing it with me or with her PCP, my mom jumped at the chance.

Being an academic medical center, in addition to the expected teams of teams, there were medical students, residents and any number of doctors-in-training. The informed consent form was a blur handled by an unnamed team member with little discussion of any risks. My mom had the surgery and was elated about the prospect of her new foot, still hidden under the surgical dressing. After a brief recovery, she was sent home with brief discharge instructions and told to follow up with the hospital in two weeks.

On her third day home, even under the dressing she could see that her repaired toe seemed to lose its beautiful alignment. She called the surgeon's office but they didn't seem concerned. Another day went by and now she insisted to be seen. Her surgeon was busy so she saw a fellow. When this doctor removed the dressing, my mother's toe was now angling in the opposite direction! The fellow downplayed the appearance, saying it may have come slightly loose but it would scar and come into alignment.

At that point, my mom should have called a timeout. She should have insisted to be seen by her original surgeon. Her gut said that things had gone wrong, but healthcare told her everything was okay. She trusted the wrong voice. Two weeks later with the toe practically deviating at a right angle now away from her toes, she couldn't even entertain wearing a shoe at all. When her surgeon finally saw her at the two-week follow-up, he knew immediately that the surgery had failed and asked why she hadn't called earlier! He explained that unless it was fixed again, she would have an outward-pointing toe for life. Would she let them into her foot again? No way! She was done with toe surgery. My mother has accepted her oddly shaped foot, not wanting to risk an even worse fate.

Years later her lung doctor recommended sinus surgery and an alarm went off. "No way. I am done with surgery!" she told him. My mom has chronic bronchitis and scarring in her lungs, and despite an exhaustive search the cause has eluded diagnosis. With her lung function stable, her doctor has stopped short of a lung biopsy and she seems to do just fine. Now she had developed a paralyzed vocal cord, making her voice barely audible. Maybe sinus surgery could jump-start the cord and free up her breathing too? She asked me about the sinus surgery and I recommended a second opinion. The second ear, nose, and throat (ENT) doctor agreed with the first that the sinus surgery could help her sinuses, her lungs, and possibly her voice, with drainage and constant infections playing a role in both.

This time her ENT went carefully through all the risks and benefits of surgery and my mom asked every doctor on the team for his or her opinion. Everyone including her PCP approved of the treatments strategy. The surgery went off without a hitch, and she has never been better. Her voice is back to normal and her lungs are going strong. I tell this tale of two surgeries to caution anyone faced with these decisions: the right surgery can put your health back on track, but the wrong surgery can send it careening off the rails.

Actually, three things can happen when you have surgery and two of them are bad. The same has been said of a throwing play in the NFL—when you put the ball in the air, three things can happen and two of them are bad! The good thing, of course, is to catch the ball. An interception and dropping the ball are the other two things that could happen, neither of which is good. Similar is true when you elect to have a surgery. On the downside of surgery, you could end up worse or the same. In light of the risk and cost of surgery, both of these outcomes should be considered bad. Of course, everyone hopes instead to end up better after surgery, but like footballs that fly and bounce unpredictably, it doesn't always work out that way. I knew of a patient with severe asthma who was scheduled to undergo a five-hour back pain procedure with full anesthesia...until the anesthesiologist said no and insisted on a shorter procedure with a local anesthetic that would be less likely to provoke the patient's asthma. And after the surgery, the patient's pain wasn't any better. More often than doctors like to admit, even a quick sideline route can end up incomplete or, even worse, going the other way for a pick-six.

So when it comes to surgery, the most important choice is whether to have it at all. The decision comes down to risks and benefits. How necessary is the surgery? What if you have it? What if you don't? Let's look at some extremes to illustrate the point.

## Need: Ruptured Appendix

Imagine that one second is left in a football game. Your team is on your own forty-yard line and down by five points. If you don't throw a pass, you are almost certain to lose. This makes a pass necessary, even though there is a risk that it will be intercepted or dropped. The potential benefits are worth the risks. A running play could miraculously work as well, but the odds are extremely small. In healthcare, sometimes we are in critical situations, and the risks of the surgery really don't matter because the risk of not having surgery is so grave. Clear-cut emergencies such as a ruptured appendix are almost non-decisions. Obviously, you will choose surgery, and you are at the mercy of whatever surgeon is available. Here's one way to look at it: The risk of not having surgery is a 99 percent chance of death. There is also a two percent risk of complications. The benefit is a 97 percent chance of saving your life and the risk-benefit analysis clearly favors having surgery.

## Not Needed: Stress Fracture Spine

Older patients and especially women with more brittle bones or osteoporosis are at risk for spine and other fractures. These fractures can be very painful. Several years ago, a procedure was developed that uses cement to fix small breaks. Studies showed the procedure helps alleviate pain. The procedure took off and I, along with everyone else, started admitting patients to the hospital for this procedure. The supposed benefit was pain reduction. But the studies had only been tested on one team of patients, all with the same problem, and the studies asked this one team about their pain reduction without comparing the benefit to patients who hadn't had the procedure. When a new study randomized patients to this cement treatment or injection with harmless salt water, they found that treatment benefit was due to placebo effect and not the cement itself. In this case, we thought that the small risk of the procedure was balanced by the benefit of pain reduction. But once the dust settled on these studies, it turned out that almost zero benefit couldn't justify even the procedure's small risk.

Good surgeons will help you work through the risk-benefit calculation of a surgery you are considering. Your surgeon should also be able to cite the evidence behind his or her opinion. Ask how these studies were done. Ask if the patients in these studies were like you, with your same health challenges.

Then ask if your surgeon's opinion could possibly be influenced by a conflict between TEAM and "me"—if your surgeon is financially incentivized to perform surgery, can you be sure that his or her advice is impartial? Move forward only once you are comfortable that the quality of the information you receive makes it clear that the benefit still outweighs the risk.

## Want: Cosmetic Facelift

Imagine it's second down with ten seconds left in the first half. Your team is down by a touchdown, with the ball on the fifty-yard line. Your options are pass, run, or do nothing and let the clock run out. Unlike in the first example, you don't need to throw a pass, but you may want to take the risk of a pass in hopes of getting down the field for a quick field goal before the end of the half. In most but not all cases, facelifts are like this "want" but not "need" football decision. Rather than worrying about the risk of not having surgery (as is removing a ruptured appendix), the risk-benefit calculation is based only on the possible risks of the facelift compared to the possible benefit to your appearance or psyche. Letting time expire on the first half doesn't mean you're going to lose the football game. Deciding to not have a facelift doesn't mean you are going to die. So make sure you understand the risks. And beware when TEAM/me don't align— if your source for understanding these risks has different goals and incentives than you, consider a second opinion.

## When the Risk-Benefit Is Complex or Unclear

In reality most of your surgery decisions don't fit into the neat boxes above. A surgery won't be as obviously necessary as removal of a ruptured appendix, nor will it be as unnecessary as a treatment that proves to have no benefit. To help you with the decision-making process, ask your PCP a simple question: What will happen if I *don't* have surgery?

Sometimes, there are nonsurgical ways to treat your problem. With less risk (and possibly less reward), it's like calling a running play. Your PCP may need more tests or the opinions of specialists to help answer this question. If the nonsurgical options (including doing nothing) are unacceptable to you, then you should see a surgeon. That doesn't mean that you should have surgery—it just means that it is worth consulting with a surgeon to explore the option further.

Remember there is such a thing as too much healthcare, whether it is surgery or tests or taking medications. Overusing healthcare costs more, offers the opportunity for error, and can make your body less able to combat conditions on its own. With everything in healthcare and especially when it comes to surgery, always remember to ask, "Do I need this?"

## How to Choose a Surgeon

After several months of itching, a very good family friend visited her doctor who ordered an ultrasound. The diagnosis: bile duct cancer. Due to the lack of symptoms, this tumor is generally found late and in advanced stages. Our friend was fortunate to have caught it relatively early but would need a very complicated surgery called a "Whipple." This is one of the most complex and risky surgeries in existence. She met the surgeon her doctor recommended and was about to have the surgery.

When we talked, I called a timeout. I knew there was a surgeon who had done more Whipples than anyone in the city and he had just moved to our hospital with his partner. Our friend agreed to see him for a second opinion and ended up loving this more experienced team. They did her Whipple not only successfully but in record time, which makes the procedure much safer. She has had a total cure. The other surgeon had done about two of these procedures per year and the surgeon I knew had done more than 350, more than 20 a year. I'm not saying that the first surgeon would have botched the Whipple…but with our friend's life literally on the line, both from her cancer and from the risks of the surgery, why go with anyone but the proven best bet? But it's not just volume—a recent study showed that the more specialized a surgeon was in a certain kind of surgery, the better the outcomes for cancer and cardiac surgeries.

When you are asleep on an operating table you are literally in the hands of your surgeon. The surgeon's diagnostic ability no longer matters. It's his or her technical skill, experience, and training that count. The first step in choosing a surgeon is to check with your insurance company. The hospital where your surgery will be covered may already be chosen for you, leaving you with a much smaller pool of surgeons to choose from. For a non-complex surgery, that may be as far as you need to go— just ask the in-network hospital to assign you a surgeon.

If you have a complex problem requiring very special surgery this is only a starting point. You may have to go out of network for the best option, making cost a major concern. Be aware of the costs, but also be aware of the possible benefit of having the best surgical care. If there's a wide range of surgery outcomes, very little data describing surgical outcomes, or if the procedure has a small success rate, take into account the benefit of working with the best.

Try asking your PCP which surgeon he or she would choose to operate on their mother. Ask nurses that work in your prospective hospital—they often know the best surgeons. Don't be afraid to get several opinions. Consider whether your surgeon might have any biases and if there's a thumb on the scale either for or against the surgical option, get another, unbiased opinion. Good doctors welcome second opinions.

Here are some questions that can help you find the best surgeon:

1. How does a surgeon's success rate compare with local and national averages?
2. How many of these surgeries has the surgeon performed? How many in the past year?
3. What is the surgeon's rate of complications—for example, rates of infection?
4. How many patients die from the surgery? This is the surgeon's mortality rate.
5. Outside the established definition of "success," does the surgeon think that the procedure will help you reach your goals?
6. Who will be doing the surgery: the surgeon, a trainee, or a robot?
7. Who will handle any problems that come up after surgery?
8. How long has the surgeon's operating-room team been working together?
9. Is the surgeon board certified? What kind of training does he or she have for this specific surgery?

## Choosing a Surgery Center

More than two-thirds of all surgeries in the U.S. are performed in outpatient ambulatory surgery centers. Like freestanding emergency rooms, these facilities are like operating rooms outside of a hospital. After the very tragic death of Joan Rivers during a procedure at a surgery center, these centers must now be accredited and must report quality measures on Hospital-comapre.gov. If they fail to report, they lose 2 percent of their Medicare billing.

In Florida, all centers are listed in a centralized website with summary information relevant to their outcomes. I recently visited the site and with a few clicks was able to find a complaint filed against one of these centers, with all the official investigation paperwork available. Knowing when and how a surgical center has dropped the ball is important information if you're considering having your procedure there! Most important, in my opinion, is looking at a center's case volume. If a center is only doing a couple of these procedures a year, pick another with more experience.

Older and/or more complex patients will want their surgeries at the hospital, which will be more equipped to handle complications. Here are some questions to ask when choosing where to have your surgery:

1.  Who will be administering the anesthesia?
2.  Have we gone over all the potential risks?
3.  What are all the possible risks and benefits?
4.  Does the hospital or center have a specific surgery floor that takes care of your surgeon's patients?
5.  Does the surgeon follow a specific checklist before surgery? If so, what's on the list?

In the end, trust your gut. If you don't feel comfortable with a surgeon, find another. Trust is a key component for all teams and you must trust the person who is cutting you open and closing you back up. In an ideal world, your dream surgeon would be extremely skilled, experienced, and brilliant, and would have good bedside manner. If you have to compromise, forget the bedside manner—you probably won't remember much of your time with this person, anyway. Once you have a surgeon and she has told you all the relevant benefits and risks, go back to your PCP to review it all. Remember that your goals and preferences are what matter the most in judging what would count as a successful surgery.

# CHAPTER 20:
## Staying Safe in Surgery

In December 2006, Raymond Grove had complex heart surgery at a hospital in Bellingham, Washington. When his surgeon left for vacation during the holiday season, Raymond's care was handed off to the hospital team. He got a new interim head coach and because Raymond had complications from his aggressive, six-hour surgery, this hospitalist managed a handful of specialists. Raymond was on a breathing tube for four days. Despite being on antibiotics, he developed what seemed to be an infection in his left leg. His calf was swollen, red, and painful to the touch and he had weakness when bending his ankle. By now, Raymond had started very basic physical therapy but was dragging his left toe when he tried to walk.

To the team of doctors and specialists, it looked like cellulitis, a bacterial infection.

However, it turned out that Raymond didn't have a bacterial infection. He had something called "compartment syndrome"—basically, a massive buildup of pressure in the compartment of his left calf muscle. One reason he was misdiagnosed is that Raymond didn't complain of the excruciating pain that is a defining symptom of compartment syndrome… but he had been on heavy pain meds since his surgery, which might have masked his calf pain.

By the time Raymond was correctly diagnosed and underwent another surgery to relieve compartment syndrome, it was too late. He had suffered irreversible muscle loss in his leg, resulting in a permanent injury. Raymond sued for malpractice and won his first case, with the jury awarding him $583,000 in damages. But then a higher court reversed the ruling on appeal. Here's the important part: the judge in this case ruled that while the team had failed, no one person on that team could be held negligent, writing that "the plaintiff is still required to prove negligence on the part of the particular employee. A team isn't negligent," and instead there needed "to be a negligent player on the team."

Due to misdiagnosis and mistreatment, Raymond Grove left the hospital with a permanent limp. But because it was a team breakdown without any single bad actor, who could he sue? Without one person to point the finger at, how could Raymond seek justice for his botched surgery experience?

I spoke with Mr. Grove's attorney, Kevin Keefe, who filled me in on the end of the story. After first winning and then losing twice, the Washington State Supreme Court ruled in favor of Mr. Grove, writing that a member of the team didn't meet the standard of care in monitoring for compartment syndrome. This is important: rather than somehow finding a way to hold the team responsible for medical malpractice, the Washington State Supreme Court remained required to find one person to hold accountable for the mistake. Once they found this person but not before, the court was able to rule in Raymond's favor.

Teams are the future of healthcare and I believe that if managed carefully, teams hold great promise, allowing each person to bring his or her specialty to the table. Teams hold great promise. But they also hold great danger. According to *Harvard Business Review,* in 2015, 65 million surgeries were performed in the U.S. with an estimated 200,000 deaths from complications. Of course, many of these deaths were due to complicated surgeries with expected mortalities. And advances in technologies and procedures are pushing this rate lower than it has been in past years. For example, laproscopic and other techniques of less invasive surgery often come with lower rates of complications. On the process side, there is a push to standardize every step of surgery, as if a surgical procedure was the equivalent of a car being built in an advanced factory. Hospitals have even been measured on some of these standardized steps, with results reported on hospitalcompare.gov. These advances have helped but errors remain.

In a *Harvard Business Journal* article exploring surgery complication rates, Dr. Atul Gawande says, "what distinguishes the great from the mediocre is not that they failed less. They rescued more." Think of a fumble in the NFL. Some teams fumble more but recover most of them. In 2015, the Patriots recovered all their fumbles. In medicine, it is usually another member of the team that has the situational awareness to be in the right place at the right time to anticipate and "recover" situations that could otherwise cause harm. This team member must react fast and without hesitation to jump on the ball.

I remember practicing fumble drills for hours. The first thing you do when you see a fumble is to communicate with your team. Everyone yells, "Fumble!" If problems arise after your surgery you want the team reacting the same way: Fast and effective communication with each other to get your care back on track.

Think about the stories you've heard in this book. In most cases, unfortunate outcomes haven't been the result of botched surgeries, but failed care afterward. Surgery sets the stage, but it's the inability of a team to recognize and repair a fumble *after* surgery that makes it dangerous. Complications will inevitably arise. Many studies on surgical quality have found the response to a complication is where the balls are dropped.

Think about the young man who developed a migraine after chemotherapy that turned out to be a brain bleed rather than a simple headache. Think about my mom whose misaligned toe was left too long. Think about Raymond, whose surgery went as well as expected but led to mismanaged complications.

One model for catching and fixing surgical problems, being piloted by Johns Hopkins and the University of Michigan, is called PERFECT, or "Perioperative Enhancement of Rescue by Fostering Engagement, Communication and Teamwork." This groundbreaking model is explained in detail on their website, Improvingrescue.com, and assesses key elements such as teamwork, communication, respect, and leadership necessary for effective rescue from major postsurgical complications. As heartening as it is to see efforts underway to fix the problem of surgery fumbles, I think this model still leaves an important player off the team, namely *you*. It's not that you are or should be responsible for your own safety during surgery, but there are certainly things you can and should do to keep the other players on track. Here are some of the things you can do to keep yourself safe during and after surgery:

## Who Is in Charge?

As in the case of Mr. Grove and his misdiagnosed compartment syndrome, make sure you know who is ultimately responsible for your care. This can be difficult when there are doctors and surgeons and anesthesiologists and nutritionists and medical students and nurses and residents and more coming in and out of your room. Still, the buck stops with somebody and it's essential to know who that person is. After surgery, your surgeon will usually be your attending, or main, physician. As you wake from surgery to find yourself in the recovery room, don't hesitate to ask, "Who is the attending on my case?" Your PCP or hospitalist may still see you, but your surgeon or the "attending" surgeon is officially now in charge. This person will write the main orders like when you can eat or walk or go home. Make sure the name of your attending is written on your hospital room white board. If your attending changes, make sure the change is noted on the board. If you stay in the hospital after your surgery is healed, responsibility for your care may transfer back to your PCP or hospitalist. Again, this change should be reflected on your whiteboard. If you lose track of who is ultimately in charge of your care, ask your nurse.

## Beware Instant Handoffs

My sister needed surgery on her uterus but she is a busy attorney and only had a small window in her schedule. Her favorite surgeon was available in this window, but was leaving for a ski trip the next morning. I advised her to reschedule—there was no need to rush her procedure. Knowing my sister, I should have known she would go ahead anyway. Her surgery went well and off went her surgeon on his trip, handing off her recovery to another surgeon associated with the hospital. Sorry to say it, but this guy was a jerk. Not only was he rude and dismissive, but he missed a nick that turned into an abscess, landing my sister in the hospital for 14 days with a catheter in her bladder. Would the team have recovered this fumble had the original surgeon stayed on her case? I think the chances are pretty good the answer is yes.

## Beware Robots

Not even the football practice dummy is immune to the technological revolution. Five NFL teams are now using robot dummies developed at Dartmouth College. These remote-controlled tackling robots are on wheels and can turn and cut and even go faster than an NFL player. Check them out on YouTube. Like the robot receiver, medicine is increasingly turning to robots to replace a surgeon's hands and scalpel. New tools like laparoscopes have made surgery much less invasive and, in the end, safer, allowing surgeons to make a tiny cut to access surgery sites with the robot's tiny arms rather than the large cut needed for a human surgeon. But it's worth noting your surgeon's use of robots. Some surgeries are more and less successful with robots. Some surgeons have more or less experience with them. Before you opt for robot-assisted surgery, look at the studies done on this type of robot and what your surgeon's training and statistics are on the machine. What part of the surgery will the robot do and what will the surgeon do?

What are the possible complications with the particular robot and how will the surgeon step in to handle these complications?

## Check Complication and Infection Rates

In October 2014, all elective surgeries at Mission Hospital, the third-largest hospital in Orange County, California, were put on hold after four patients who underwent orthopedic operations developed infections. In other words, infections and complications at the hospital-wide level are not just a hypothetical—they're real and you don't want your surgery at a place where they happen.

Check the Joint Commission website and Hospitalcompare.gov for red flags. However, it can take weeks or months or more for a hospital's challenges to show up on these government sites and so it's also worth a Google search to see if there's late-breaking news about your hospital. If you find red flags, talk to your surgeon. Your surgeon should be able to tell you what's being done about any problems.

## Recover on the Right Floor

Hospitals have specialized recovery areas for different types of surgeries, including cardiac, neurologic, orthopedic, and others. Nurses and hospitalists in these wards are experienced with the types of recovery needs and complications patients tend to have after these surgeries. But not all surgery patients get to recover in their hospital's specialized area! If there are no empty beds in the hospital, spaces in the specialized recovery wards can go to non-surgical patients. Or emergencies and other unplanned events can push around your plan. This process of bed assignment can be more complicated than air control at JFK. Hospitals try to make the best decisions based on what is best for most—but this is an example of a TEAM/me conflict in which what's best for the hospital is not necessarily best for you. On another floor, your surgeon will still watch over your recovery, but the rest of the team might not be as experienced. Talk to your team ahead of time to discuss how certain it is that you will be allowed to recover on the ward designated for your surgery. If the chance isn't what you hope, you might reconsider your choice of hospital. As always, if your concerns aren't answered, call a timeout!

## Surgery Game Plan

You've seen the elements of good game P.L.A.N.S. Now let's see how this looks with surgery:

- ▶ **Patient Centered:** Make sure based on your goals and preferences that having surgery is worth the risk and that the surgeon knows the outcomes you desire. Make sure your team knows your definition of success so that everyone on the team can help make decisions that point toward this goal.
- ▶ **Learning:** Learn all you can about the risks and benefits of surgery. Then learn all you can about the surgeons you are considering and if you have any doubts at all, get second and third opinions. Learn about what you need to do before and after surgery to maximize your chance of success. On the hospital side, help your team learn about you and what your expectations are.
- ▶ **Assignments:** Before, during, and after your surgery, you and the team will have assignments. For example,

some surgeries will benefit from rehab or exercise before the surgery. During your stay, your assignments may include walking as soon as possible or using your incentive spirometer to prevent pneumonia. Your surgeon will have assignments as a coach and as a player, and everyone on the hospital team will have assignments based on your needs.

▶ **Notify:** Remember, not all surgery complications can be prevented, but with quick recognition and care, many can be prevented from turning into big problems. Some of this responsibility is yours. There's likely to be some discomfort after surgery, but don't be tough. If you experience signs and symptoms that seem more or different than expected, notify your team right away. Then you may have to make sure that your team notifies other important team members. Unfortunately, in the hospital, what people don't know can kill you.

▶ **Success:** Before surgery, you defined your criteria for success and now it's time to measure them. At your follow-up appointment, talk with your surgeon about how and whether the procedure has helped you meet your goals. If your goals have not been met, there will need to be a new game plan to achieve them. This plan may include additional work with your surgeon or may better be accomplished with your PCP or another specialist. Best case scenario and with these guidelines in mind, you can make your surgery a touchdown!

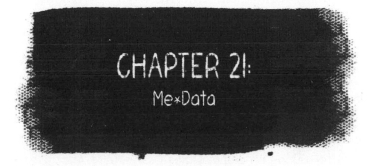

# CHAPTER 21:
## Me*Data

Michael practically lived on a plane. The constant grind was tough but so was the job market and traveling paid the bills. The realities of his schedule meant that Michael skipped many doctor visits but he was only in his late 40s and was healthy...except for a small hole in his heart. He'd been diagnosed years ago and it never gave him any trouble except when he failed sports physicals. In fact, Michael never thought much about it except he was supposed to get antibiotics when he got his teeth cleaned.

Now after a long week of travel and a six-hour flight home, Michael was ready for some exercise the next morning. His wife and children were out of town for a birthday and he had a rare chance to ride his mountain bike, which sat lonely in the corner of his garage. His left leg was swollen and slightly red but that was not going to stop this long overdue ride. About an hour into the ride on a picturesque trail he suddenly veered off the path, confused by a split in the trail. He nearly crashed but was able to stop unscathed. That's when he knew something was wrong—he couldn't figure out what to do next. Suddenly, Michael was like a five-year-old riding a bike for the first time. He tried anyway and fell hard. His thoughts grew hazy and splintered like the light through the massive trees.

Luckily that's when a couple biked up the trail behind him. By that point, Michael couldn't talk; he just stared at the couple, bewildered. The couple called 911 and after a quick evacuation, Michael was rushed to the ER.

Now, you know Michael's health history, but here's what the ER saw: late 40s male found on the side of a mountain bike trail after taking an obvious crash. Of course, they assumed he'd hit his head and worked him up with X-rays and a head CT. Michael's cell phone was locked and he wasn't carrying identification. Given his confusion there was nothing Michael could do to flesh out the picture—no way for the ER to know about his medical history and the hole in his heart. Sure, his left leg was a little red and swollen, but it seemed easily explained by the bike crash.

Michael's CT scan was negative but they kept him for observation and at about 3:00 am that morning, he was able to unlock his phone and a nurse helped him call his wife. Michael was still not able to communicate clearly and so the nurse filled in his wife, telling her that Michael had crashed his mountain bike and hit his head. Michael's wife was so relieved he was okay and, with the information she had, was confident that Michael was recovering from what was obviously a bad concussion, that she didn't mention anything about Michael's health history.

At 5:00 am the nurse came in to take Michael's vital signs but couldn't shake him awake. He was not responding, drooling from the side of his mouth, which was drooping to one side. His entire body slumped to the right. The nurse called a stroke alert. He was rushed to the CT scanner and then to the ICU—a massive stroke had knocked out half his brain. The doctors tried to stabilize him as they ordered an EKG of his heart and ultrasound of his leg. There were the real causes of his confusion and swollen leg: a blood clot in his leg and the hole in his heart. The doctors gave Michael clot-busting medication but his condition worsened. As his wife got on a plane, Michael went onto a ventilator. She arrived just before he died as the swelling overtook his brain.

Michael knew his past medical history but his team did not. If the ER doctors had known he had a hole in his heart that allowed a clot in his leg to go right to his brain causing a mini-stroke on the bike trail, they could have treated him before he had the bigger, fatal stroke in the hospital. Your medical history is a story that can save your life, but only if your healthcare team knows it.

For some people, a health history is a long and complex novel and for others it is a short story. Either way, it's always evolving as every doctor you visit adds to the story. Where does the story live? Before electronic medical records, your health history was in paper charts in hospitals and doctors' offices. The problem was that in the middle of the night, there was no way for a doctor to access it. Patients had to tell their stories from memory, like ancient storytellers at a campfire at the mouth of their prehistoric cave. What if, like Michael, a patient couldn't tell the story? What then? This lead to frantic paper chases in the middle of the night with phone calls to hospitals and faxed illegible records that came slowly if they came at all. We would literally play charades with patients. We would hear things like, "Doc they took something out of my stomach and tied it to my bowel!" Was it your gallbladder or your duodenum...maybe the pancreas?

With paper health records, information routinely fell through the gaps in a way that seemed ridiculous to industries like banking that had moved to electronic record keeping. Patients began keeping their own version of the story by getting paper copies of all their records. They even made their own summaries of their story, some very detailed and others just a list of their medications. They knew the value this had to their healthcare team. Despite these efforts, a patient's DIY health record could be inaccurate or could quickly become outdated. Patient-generated information was notoriously suspect.

During my residency in 1993, I carried a pocket *Physician's Desk Reference* or PDR. It was the early stages of the med-tech revolution and the 900-page book of medications had been condensed into a small handheld computer. Amazing! It even had a file for entering data and I began to enter all my patients and their labs into my little handheld device. But I soon realized it took much longer to enter all these names and numbers into this small device than it did to write the info on notecards, like the other doctors.

I also remember when my outpatient practice got its first electronic medical record system or EMR in the late 1990s. The resistance to this new system was palpable and whether it was due to resistance or a bad system, the result was chaos. It was so bad that I started a company making handheld devices that doctors could use at the point of care with patients. Our first model weighed more than 10 pounds and looked like the stone tablet that Fred Flintstone used in the quarry. Instead of being at the "leading edge" of technology, I was at the "bleeding edge" meaning that without streamlined iPads or other less cumbersome tablets, the company was doomed. That said, I learned much from that failure. We talked of walking around with smartphones connected to the internet as a dream that has now come into reality.

Another reality is that today more than 85 percent of hospitals and 50 percent of offices have electronic medical records (EMRs) or computerized records. I have lived with many hospitals through the pain of converting from their paper systems, and trust me, it can be very scary. One hospital did it all at once, calling it the Big Bang. It was a bang alright, leading to total anarchy with doctors unable to get their lists of patients and losing track of them sometimes for days. Some older doctors simply decided to retire. It felt like the final play in the famous Stanford-Cal game when the band ran onto the field as the time ran out and nobody knew what was happening. Nurses and doctors and pharmacists tried to do their jobs in a frustrated fugue state.

Fast-forward and we have made progress but are still not where we need to be. There are still safety issues with EMRs. One issue is the difference between "big data" and the little data that is yours and yours along, which I call Me*Data.

Healthcare is trying to cure everything from cancer to colds using big data and with medical records online, there's a new boom of data available. But it's the Me*Data that is so much more important than Big Data when it comes to you and your family. In this chapter, Michael's team didn't have his Me*Data.

The problem is that keeping track of it all can be a full-time job. Why? Because healthcare is still fragmented. Your hospital may have a different EMR system than your doctor's office, which may not interface well with your specialist in another system. Remember healthcare is made up of teams of teams and like the NHL trying to share information with the NFL, sometimes there's just no connection. Back in the 1990s, we didn't expect there to be a connection. Healthcare systems were aware of the need to make careful decisions with incomplete information and so worked hard to fill in gaps that they knew existed. Now, however, doctors can get lulled into the idea that all of their patients' information is at their fingertips. Newsflash: it's not. But doctors may now fail to recognize this and fill in the gaps.

The NFL has figured out what the U.S. healthcare system has not. Granted, the NFL has about 1,696 players and the U.S. has 320 million people to keep track of, but who is counting? When I spoke with Dr. Matthew Matava, president of the NFL Physician's Society, he pointed out that when an NFL player is injured in a game, the entire medical record is instantly available for the medical team. When a player is traded or goes to another team as a free agent, the record is completely portable and follows the player to the new team. This is the Holy Grail for American healthcare. Until it reaches this ideal, you will have to be the safety on your healthcare team. Here is how.

## Organizing Your Personal Health Record

Experts who make Personal Health Record or PHR systems define them as "an electronic application used by patients to maintain and manage their health information in a private, secure, and confidential environment." But you can make your

PHR anything you want. Obviously, a PHR should include your medical information, but can also include your insurance and financial information, or even wellness information including nutrition, fitness, and sleep. Your PHR can be something you organize and update, or it can be a system managed by your employer, doctor, hospital, or insurer. Here are some things that should go in your PHR: list of medical conditions, past major procedures and illnesses, past hospitalizations, list of doctors and specialists, allergies, family medical history, history of behavior health including smoking, alcohol and drugs, your activity level and exercise, immunizations, lab and other test results, do-not-resuscitate or other end-of-life preferences, your family members and other at-home caregivers, and especially your medications.

Even if you're generally healthy and don't anticipate any major healthcare needs in the near future, I suggest keeping a PHR-light (much different than a PBR Light, which is not especially beneficial to your health!). At the very least, it should include your allergies, immunization records, and as much as you know about your family history that could guide proactive healthcare decisions like cancer screenings.

As you can see, you have to be really motivated to gather the information for your PHR yourself! The good news is that you don't necessarily have to. Most of this information, you can simply access and correct if needed. The most common place to store and manage your PHR is with your primary care physician's office. Talk with your PCP about what options are available—can the office import information directly from your pharmacy? Can their system interface with your hospital or with specialists' offices? What sort of wellness tracking systems do they automatically include or could they possibly include with your PHR? If you don't like the answers, you better bet there's an app for that. Rather than trying to reinvent the wheel in a basement filing cabinet or with files upon files upon files sitting on your computer hard drive, consider exploring the many publicly available PHR systems, some paid and some free. Some of these web- and app-based PHR systems will pull information directly from other health information sources. Some even include the option for consultation directly through their interface, allowing you to talk with a patient coordinator or other healthcare concierge. The benefit of having your own PHR is that it is your own. The problem is that it is your own. You will need to make sure it is secure and sharable. Most have a way to add members of the team that can access your record, like your family and doctors. I can't tell you how many times friends and family members, instead of trying to explain a health problem, grant me access to PHRs so that I can look at the info myself.

Then remember, if you're doing it yourself, keep it up to date. With PHRs, it's "garbage in, garbage out" meaning that if you're lax with the information that goes into your PHR, it can be useless or even dangerous when a healthcare team uses it as the basis for important decisions.

As you've seen, just as important as *having* a PHR is making sure it's accessible to your healthcare team. If Michael had used an app that allowed the emergency room team to access a PHR stored on his phone, he might still be alive today. Even if you don't put your whole PHR on your phone, consider adding just your "In Case of Emergency" or ICE plan to it. Instructions for how to add ICE to your phone are an easy Google search away. Or you can go the route of one of my colleagues, Casey Quinlan, who got a QR code tattooed on her chest that scans to her advanced directives in her PHR. She learned from her father's battle with Parkinson's disease and his graceful death to document her wishes early and often. In her father's case, healthcare wanted to give him a feeding tube but Casey said no, at peace with her decision because her father had spelled out his wishes more than a decade earlier.

This entire movement of letting patients look into their medical records grew from a concept called Open Notes, in which patients could not only access, but edit and correct their PHRs. A pilot study at world-renowned Geisinger Medical Center found that 89 percent of patients who had access to their medical records requested corrections to these records. In a similar study at the VA only 5 percent of the time did the computer medication record match up with what the patient said they were taking. In other words, the Open Notes movement let patients double-check that healthcare's understanding of their lives matched the real world. The new direction of the Health Information Technology both from policy and business standpoints is toward this open integration of information in which doctors and hospitals ensure that information flows smoothly to a centralized record and then patients are able to access this record to consult it and correct it as needed. The best part of this kind of PHR is it literally puts you and your healthcare team on the same page of your story—you are doing what the PHR says and the PHR says what you're doing.

Perhaps closest to this ideal PHR system is Kaiser Permanente's "My Care Manager." When your insurer and your doctors and your hospitals and your specialists and your pharmacists are all on the same team, then your PHR can be a one-stop shop. From the My Care Manager website you can: send a message or email your doctor's office, track your insurance spending and pay bills, use the pharmacy, see your medical record, make an appointment, and access patient education or learning sites. If you get care from only one doctor's office or hospital system, you might similarly be able to organize and access most or all of your health information from the system's portal.

Consider starting your PHR search at myPHRsearch.com or HealthIT.gov and keep the following in mind: If you make your own PHR, make sure it is accurate and up-to-date; try to use existing systems from your doctor, hospital, insurer or employer; even if you use a pre-built, supposedly automatic PHR, check in frequently to make sure there are no errors; keep an eye out for new PHR products from these institutional sources or from startups—Health Information Technology is one of the fastest-evolving of all sectors and what's best today is almost certain to be eclipsed by something better tomorrow.

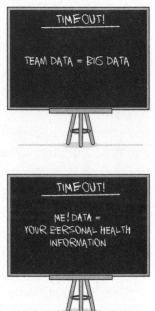

# Section Three
## Troubleshooting the Bill

A s a resident, I worked grueling hours, even getting lost while driving home once after being awake more than 36 hours. One night during my neurology rotation, the senior resident was home getting some much-needed rest and I was called to see a patient with sudden weakness of her arm and one side of her face—obvious signs of a stroke. I ordered a CT to get a clear diagnosis, but the nurse also alerted me to her blood pressure, which was high and climbing. At the same time, I was called on two other patients, one who was developing a life-threatening infection and another who was showing signs of meningitis. Pulled in three directions, I made my first mistake: I didn't call for help. As a matter of pride, I didn't want to wake up my senior resident. I could handle it!

Before taking care of the patients with infection and meningitis, I gave my stroke patient medication to reduce her blood pressure. Finally, I thought I was all caught up...until the nurse called to tell me the stroke patient's blood pressure was now dangerously low! I rushed to the floor and gave her IV fluid to bolster her blood pressure, but it remained very low. During this time, her stroke extended and got much bigger. Finally, I called the senior resident. The next day, the patient had started improving, but there was no doubt that I had made things worse.

Believe me, I beat myself up way more than my professors did. I remember apologizing to the patient and explaining what had happened, but she had no family and given her advanced age and now with the influence of the stroke, she didn't really understand. As she improved, I beat myself up less but found myself double- and triple-checking my orders. I needed to forgive myself to help my current and future patients—when you're in crunch time, you can't have fear ruling your decisions. Finally, the old adage "forgive but don't forget" allowed me to move on. I learned to ask for help early and often and I never dropped another stroke patient's blood pressure.

Now I have used this story to teach many other residents and doctors. We don't usually walk around eager to tell our worst stories of failure, but let me tell you, most doctors can recount their worst mistakes in excruciating detail—they're much more top-of-mind than our greatest cures. All this is to show that doctors make mistakes. We do the best damn job we possibly can, but we're still fallible. The truly unfortunate part is that our mistakes can have consequences. The phrase "you win some, you lose some" is attributed to a dozen or more sports figures, especially including baseball coaches like Yogi Berra and Sparky Anderson. But while it might be okay to lose a baseball game, there's no room for this kind of thinking in medicine. When it's a matter of life and death, you can't just happen to "lose some."

And still, some get lost.

This section is about what to do when healthcare goes wrong—when you get an unexpected bill or need to negotiate the cost of your care.

# CHAPTER 22:
## OOPs! Dealing With Surprise Out-of-Pocket Spending

Kelly struggled to balance the demands of her job with being the mother of three thriving children. Meals in the car on the way to soccer and gymnastics and homework on the baseball diamond were her life—and she wouldn't have had it any other way. Single mothers don't get vacation days, even when they are sick. Kelly didn't have time for the pain in her chest, hoping it would work itself out, like her back aches had a couple years ago. One morning just as her daughter jumped into her bed, the pain came on like a vice grip, her kids startled by her scream. Kelly called her mother who told her to dial 911.

Instead, without helping hands for the kids, Kelly tossed them in the car and asked her mother to meet her at the hospital around the corner. They got there at the same time and Kelly was rushed into the back as her mother comforted the children. Kelly knew from her mother's heart disease this could be bad. She was only 40, but exercise and good nutrition had fallen by the wayside after her divorce and she counted smoking as a guilty pleasure, her only stress relief.

It turned out that Kelly was not having a heart attack, but the ER doctor worried about a developing blockage and called a cardiologist into the case. The cardiologist wanted more info on Kelly's heart function and scheduled a cardiac catheterization—a procedure in which a thin tube is inserted into the blood vessel leading to the heart to find possible blockages. This meant that Kelly needed to be admitted to the hospital, which had her worried on so many levels. "What about the kids' teacher conferences and the dog?" she thought. She also worried what it would mean for her and her family if she did, in fact, have heart damage. She had her catheterization late that night and was finally taken to a hospital room at about three in the morning. When she woke the next morning, her cardiologist told her that the catheterization had found some blockages, which they had been able to clear. "You have new plumbing!" he said. They talked about changes she would need to make, including stopping smoking and taking care of her health. In all, Kelly ended up staying in the hospital for three days.

The last thing on Kelly's mind was insurance and networks and deductibles. She had never fully read her company's benefit book, but the hospital was in network. What was there to worry about? Two weeks later, the bill arrived. It was a stretch, but she paid her part. Then another bill arrived. It turned out that while the hospital was in network, the doctors were not. The hospital told her that her insurance company should cover the out-of-network doctors because her treatment was considered emergency care. She called her insurance company and after enough time to memorize their on-hold music, the insurer offered to pay a much lower fee—one that the hospital doctors refused to accept. The hospital pointed at the insurance company. The insurance company pointed at the doctors. The doctors wanted to be paid for their work. And Kelly was lost in the middle, alone.

Surprise out-of-pocket spending or "OOPs" is the new bombshell of medical care. A 2013 study found that 40 percent of patients who incurred out-of-network fees did so expecting their care to be in-network, and every year 30 percent of privately insured patients are hit with surprise bills. A Kaiser Family Foundation poll found that 7 out of 10 patients who visited an out-of-network provider thought the provider was in-network at the time of care. As insurers continue to narrow their networks to reduce costs and providers choose carefully which policies they do and do not accept, there will only be more potential for OOPs in the years to come. The Kaiser Family Foundation notes that about a quarter of U.S. adults say they or someone in their house has had problems paying medical bills in the past 12 months. And economists debate whether medical bills are the number one or number two cause of bankruptcies.

Have you had an unexpected envelope arrive in the mail a couple weeks after using healthcare? The first step to avoiding these OOPs is knowing where they come from.

## Where Do OOPs! Come From?

OOPs! happen when patients are caught between teams of teams, in the disconnect between where treatment happens (hospital or facility), the people who provide treatment (doctors and specialists), and the entities that pay for care (insurance companies). Unfortunately, it's kind of like working with an ice skating arena, an NFL coach, and a municipal government to figure out who should pay for stadium air conditioning. If everyone were on the same team, as can be the case in HMO systems like Kaiser, it would be easy—you go to the team hospital where the team doctors work and are covered by the team insurance. Good luck finding that with your employer's private insurance plan at your local hospital!

Outside HMOs, the network of care is like an NFL owner negotiating individual contracts with each stadium and coach. This results in a tangled web in which doctors can work in a hospital but not be hired by the hospital. And even if you have an in-network head coach, the rest of the player-coaches like anesthesiologists and surgeons and radiologists and pathologists and even physical therapists may not be covered. These complex and disconnected agreements are where patients get stuck. Why? Because, in an emergency, these out-of-network facilities or providers can be drafted onto the team with little regard for cost or who is paying. On one hand, that's a good thing. In this chapter, Kelly couldn't wait until she felt better to get the opinion of an in-network cardiologist. But on the other hand, being assigned a doctor or specialist is a crapshoot that can lead directly to OOPs!

Yes, your insurer is responsible for covering your emergency care, even if it is out-of-network or includes pieces that are out-of-network. But often insurance companies have negotiated in-network fees with their approved providers. These negotiated fees are likely to be less than an out-of-network doctor charges. So, for example, if you end up needing emergency eyebrow surgery and are rushed into the care of an out-of-network eyebrow surgeon, your insurance is required to pay for the procedure...but if your insurance is used to paying $1,000 and your surgeon charges $1,500, you're still on the hook for $500. This is called "balance billing" and it's a major source of OOPs!

This happens in the NFL all the time. Remember when Tim Tebow was traded from the Denver Broncos to the New York Jets? I was at the owners' meeting when it was announced and reporters swarmed Jets owner, Woody Johnson, who was excited about the deal at the time. As part of the deal, the Jets would pay the "balance" of Tebow's signing bonus—a remaining OOPs! of $1.53 million. It was as if Tebow were an expensive procedure and the difference between Jets and Broncos was that between an in-network and out-of-network provider. (Unfortunately for the Jets, the "procedure" wasn't the cure they'd hoped it would be...see this book's chapter about botched surgeries.)

Here's the thing: once you're in an emergency situation, there is really nothing you can do to avoid OOPs! in our patched-together system of individually negotiated contracts. When your life or health or wellbeing is on the line, you can't call a timeout until you can nail down an in-network provider. If possible, bring your "agent" with you—a family member or trusted friend can help sift through the expensive things you might not need. But a more successful way to avoid OOPs! is to lay the groundwork for prevention.

## The OOPs! Prevent Defense

If you did your homework in sections One and Two in the book you have already minimized your chance of getting surprise medical bills from out-of-network doctors and hospitals. You took the time as a restricted or true free agent to let your choice of doctors and hospitals drive your insurance decisions.

Before any elective or planned procedures, you checked and double-checked to make sure everyone involved was on your team. If you chose a facility outside your covered hospital, you made sure it's in network. And you made a list of in-network emergency facilities so that even for unplanned care you can at least land at a stadium in your network. That's the "prevent defense" that can help you avoid a big play against you. Great job! Now the challenge becomes what to do when your prevent defense is challenged—despite doing everything you can ahead of time, emergencies arise and when they do you can still find the opportunity for OOPs! Here are some ways to avoid OOPs even in the midst of unplanned care.

## Wear Your Jersey, Insist on Your Team

How can you know a player's team if he doesn't wear his jersey? It's the same going into the hospital or emergency room—how can the staff know what insurance team you're on unless you tell them? Sometimes that's all it takes to ensure the care you receive will be covered. I recently spoke to an important patient advocate about this and she agreed that it *should* be perfectly possible in today's age of instant information, once a hospital knows a patient's insurance, to match that patient with care that is covered by the insurance. But that's often not the case. Even when a hospital knows your insurance, you can end up with doctors and treatments that aren't covered. One reason is another example of how TEAM and "me" can misalign.

See, hospitals and doctors may be able to earn more money for treatments that are given out-of-network. This is particularly true if an insurer has negotiated a very competitive price with the in-network doctors. The reason you get stuck with out-of-network care is that hospitals and doctors may be financially incentivized to provide your care out-of-network. I'm not saying there's a conscious strategy on the part of healthcare providers to bilk patients out of their life savings by intentionally providing out-of-network care, but a hospital may not go far down their list to find an in-network option when doing so goes against its financial interests.

So, whose duty is it to tell you when care is out-of-network? The hospital or the doctor or the insurer? Until the system figures this out, I recommend you take action. Tell the patient representative when you check in that you want only care that is covered by your insurance plan. Then make sure that each head coach and interim head coach knows your wish to see only in-network specialists. For example, tell the ER doctor you would like to talk to the case manager about checking to make sure any specialists the doc wants on your case are in-network. If the ER doctor wants you to work with an out-of-network specialist because it's the only option or because the ER doc thinks a certain person is best for your case, ask that the doctor clear the choice with you beforehand.

If you're admitted, have the same conversation with your hospitalist. Before bringing a specialist on board, ask your hospitalist to have someone call the specialist's office to see if he or she takes your insurance. Trust me, this is a common phone call, but usually it's done to weed out patients on Medicaid or with no insurance at all. Why shouldn't you have the same check in the system? If a specialist is not in-network, he or she should be able to work with your hospitalist to find someone who is. Granted, you may need to go with an out-of-network choice, but by asking and working with your head coach, at least you can make this your choice and not a surprise.

## Use Your Agents

When you're using healthcare, your family members are your agents. They can do two important things: first, they can watch over your care to keep you safe and, second, they can track and document everything that happens. As doctors line up at your door, have your agents ask if they are in-network. Have your family write down doctors' names and specialties. Have them note major tests and medications. Then when you get that huge bill from the hospital, check it against this list. As my insurance reminds me on their website, four out of ten medical bills are inaccurate.

Finally, if there are complications, documenting exactly what went wrong, when and why can help you dispute parts of the bill that the hospital should cover. For example, if you get an infection or have injuries from a fall, the hospital may be responsible for some of the costs.

## Preventative Care Is Free

The ACA mandated all preventative services are supposed to be free. This means that for services designated "A" or "B" by the U.S. Preventive Services Task Force, your insurance company should pay in full—no co-pays or deductibles or anything out of your pocket. Now, determining what is on this list is where shared decision making and science and politics all come together. Remember the "need, don't need, and want" concept of choosing whether or not to have surgery? Government, healthcare, and insurance go through a similar calculus when deciding which preventive services should be free. Maybe you heard the hubbub when the USPTF recommended that women should start getting mammograms at age 50 instead of 40? One reason this was a big deal is that it set the stage for insurance companies to start refusing to pay for mammograms until patients turn 50. Because the list of free preventive care services is always changing, you'll want to search Healthcare.gov for "preventive care benefits" to see the most recent list. Some highlights include the recent addition of lung cancer screenings. If you are between the ages of 55 and 80 and are a smoker or quit within the past 15 years, you can get a free lung cancer screening CAT. Similar free screenings are offered for colon and breast cancers, and insurers may cover prostate cancer screening (PSA test) but it is not currently recommended (USPTF level D), as most men have slow, non-aggressive tumors. This makes screening less effective. Ask your doctor to discuss the pros and cons of having this test; it is a personal decision. Obesity screening and counseling is covered. Screening for hepatitis C is also covered, with the understanding that curing Hep C can potentially prevent the liver cancer associated with the disease. While you're at it, get screened for HIV and hepatitis B as well, if you are at risk. Depression screening is another free, often overlooked service. With the ACA, mental health screening and care must be covered just like physical health. Women and children are eligible for special services including well-baby visits.

Still, before taking advantage of any of these free preventive screenings and services, make sure to clarify with your doctor that these services are free and that you want the visit to be billed for that service. If you bring up any other issue during your visit, the appointment may be billed as a regular visit and not as a free screening. Also recognize that you may need to follow up your free screening with not-free confirmation tests or other procedures. For example, if you require a biopsy as part of your colonoscopy, the biopsy may not be covered. Or if your family medical history or genetic testing means that you require more frequent or earlier screenings, these might not be covered. Always clarify with your insurer ahead of time.

## When OOPs! Happen

When you're hit with OOPs!, the first thing to do is know your rights. The ACA tried to protect against some of these surprise bills, but like so many aspects of the healthcare bureaucracy, it can be a bit of a maze to figure out how the ACA's mandates affect your costs. For example, the ACA stops insurers from charging higher co-pays or co-insurance for out-of-network care (but doesn't protect against *balance billing*). Also, insurers can still require prior approval—if a procedure or medicine is covered, it is safest to check ahead of time. However, plans initiated before March 23, 2010 may be grandfathered into the ability to break these rules. And you may still have to jump through the hoop of approval for employer-based or short-term plans.

These ACA loopholes leave you vulnerable, so about a quarter of states have passed or are passing their own laws to protect you from OOPs! bills. For example, New York prohibits balance billing for out-of-network care received at an in-network facility (meaning that out-of-network providers have to accept the in-network fee). Check your state's protections before you spend time and effort fighting the bill. When I spoke with Chuck Bell, programs director for the Consumer's Union, he suggested contacting your state insurance commissioner's office to explore their protections and advocacy services.

## Watch for TEAM/Me Alliances and Conflicts

Often an OOPs! bill isn't your doctor's fault. He or she wants the insurance company to pay for your care. Only, sometimes the care your doctor orders is denied or underpaid by your insurance. In this case, consider enlisting your doctor to help you get your care covered. I have done this throughout my career, for example pushing insurance companies to cover tests they initially denied. Or sometimes a hospital will ask a doctor to include more detail describing a patient's condition so that the hospital can more fully bill the insurance company. For instance, if I write that a patient is anemic or has low blood count without noting the cause of the anemia, the insurance company may pay less than if I note that the anemia is due to blood loss.

Unfortunately, OOPs! bills can also make your team misalign. My wife once got a letter from her insurance company stating that, "Our clinical staff may contact your physician or the hospital at some point during your admission to offer assistance with discharge planning." In this case *assistance with discharge planning* is code for "we will ask your hospital to kick you out ASAP to keep costs down." Rather than working together toward the end zone, OOPs! can make the four members of the team—patient (player), doctor (coach), insurer (owner), and hospital (stadium)—line up across from each other. Unusual alliances and enemies can arise.

## What to Do With OOPs!

First make sure the OOPs! is real. Trust me, bills always seem to go out on time and find their way to your mailbox, but they're not always spot-on correct. Make sure that in addition to the bottom line, you get a complete itemized version of all your bills. Based on your deductible and co-insurance, the hospital should tell you before you go home what you will likely owe. If you see an error, call your insurer right away.

Then put your bills in three piles: hospital, doctors, and insurers. The hospital and doctors should bill your insurance company directly and so bills coming from hospitals and doctors should clearly show your insurer's part and your part. Check these hospital/doctor bills against your insurance bills. The charges on these bills should line up with the amounts your insurer says is their part.

When things don't align, start with your insurer. Because your insurer is used to disputing hospital bills, it's good to have them on your side as you dissect your OOPs! bill. Work with your insurance company to go through the list of treatments, visits and medicines to make sure everything on the bills was actually done. Did you really see all these doctors? Did you really get that medication or test, or maybe was it ordered and then cancelled...and you still got charged for it? Were you charged for an assistant surgeon to help your surgeon? Tell your insurance company about any discrepancies—you better bet your insurer will be motivated to inform the other entities on your team that there's no need to pay for mistaken billings.

Then ask which charges are due to the realities of your care and which might be due to hospital errors. I'm not saying that every bill is evidence of malpractice, but sometimes your hospital will pay for preventable complications. Sometimes hospitals will be up front about infections or falls or other accidents of care, but, unfortunately, you may still sometimes see costs associated with these hospital mistakes showing up on your bill. OOPs!

Also, check that care billed as out-of-network is, in fact, out-of-network. Wouldn't it be an easy fix to discover that your surgeon takes your insurance after all? Insurance lists can be out of date and delays and changes in doctors' insurance contracts happen all the time.

Then if the bill seems correct but your insurance denies the claim, let your insurer know immediately that you are asking for a review. This will buy some time. Let your doctor's office manager or hospital know too—this can keep the billing department from pushing to collect the bill. This breathing space gives the insurance company time to negotiate with the hospital—sometimes your insurer and hospital will be able to agree on a smaller charge for your care, dramatically reducing your OOPs!

If your insurer cannot work it out or says there is nothing they can do about your bill, go a step further than requesting a review and file a formal appeal. Again, this will buy you time and hold off any collection process. Notify the doctor's office manager, as this should hold off their attempts to collect as well. Use this time to check your state's protections. Also explain any extenuating circumstances to your doctor's office manager. If your hospital/doctor knows your situation, they might be willing to accept smaller reimbursement from your insurer. (I've done this more times than I can count.) Typically, an appeal gives you 90 days to sort everything out. If all else fails, you can contact your state insurance commissioner to ask for his/her help or to recommend a patient advocate to work with your case.

## Patient Advocates Are Professional Agents

As good as it is to have your family by your side to help watch over your care and troubleshoot your billing afterward, sometimes you need Jerry Maguire. Like Jerry, a professional patient advocate knows the system and has contacts among the key stakeholders. Before you look into hiring a patient advocate to help with your OOPs medical bills, check to see if you already have access to one through your employer.

According to Mercer's 2015 National Survey of Employer-Sponsored Health Plans, 52 percent of employers with more than 500 employees and 27 percent with greater than 10 employees offer patient advocate services. Remember to leverage your team's resources!

There are two major kinds of patient advocates, ones that can help you coordinate and facilitate medical care and another that can help you troubleshoot the financial side of healthcare. Some advocates or advocacy agencies do both. But beware: while researching this section of the book, I called more than a dozen patient advocates and most were little more than automated call centers. For a fee, these advocates will review your case but without a strong and experienced advocate willing to dig into the details of your case, you're unlikely to see much value.

On the medical side, a good patient advocate can empower patients' choices, ensure a patient is heard, streamline care by avoiding things like duplicate tests, and advise on value-based treatment decisions. For example, I chatted with Dr. Anette Tricora, who left medical practice to found Guided Patient Services in Columbus, Ohio.

"I do everything that doctors want to do, if only they had an extra 30 minutes with each patient," she says. Tricora explained that one of the important aspects of her role is to "take the baton" from the doctor, working with patients and their families to understand their diagnoses and options. Tricora told me the story of her very first client. A wonderful older woman had a terminal diagnosis but her young doctor hadn't yet informed the family or, really, the rest of the health-care team. The woman and her doctor knew she was dying, but the rest of the team carried on as if oblivious. With Tricora's help, the family was included in the knowledge of the diagnosis and they ended up making the decision to bring their mother and grandmother home, grateful for the opportunity to help her pass with dignity.

On the financial side of patient advocacy, I spoke with Anna Inglett, CEO of Putman Health Advocates, an advocacy firm based in Tampa, Florida. As a former medical billing specialist, Inglett saw firsthand the need for specialty guidance in patients' medical finances. In addition to hiring a professional when needed, Inglett's top suggestion for people trying to avoid big medical bills goes back to prevention—negotiate *before* a treatment rather than after, she says. When evaluating patient advocacy services, it's usually best to go a company that charges a percentage of the money they save for you. Like a true sports agent that is paid only if their client is paid, these reputable patient advocacy agencies only make money if they are successful in saving you money. For example, Putnam charges 25 percent of the money they save their clients. Of course, set-fee patient advocacy services exist as well, though if you choose this route, you will want to do your homework to discover exactly what you will get for your money—to avoid being taken advantage of, beware any advocacy agency that can't or won't provide a detailed list of what they will do to advocate for you!

## When OOPs! Come from Error

The last thing you want to do is pay for care that sets you back rather than moving your forward. If you or your team can catch these errors as they are happening, not only can you avoid seeing them on your bill, but you can avoid their health consequences as well. If you think an error has been made, call a timeout ASAP! For example, if you think you got the wrong medication notify your nurse immediately—in addition to working to counteract the effects of mistaken medication, your team can make sure you don't have to pay for bad meds. Likewise, if you think you had a test or procedure in error call a timeout! Make sure the error is actually an error and then, if it is, report it to multiple people including the head nurse on your floor and the hospital's patient representative. This is another example of proactive, prevent defense—by catching mistakes as they happen, you can prevent the need to troubleshoot an OOPs! bill when it shows up unexpectedly in your mailbox.

It takes time to decide how to proceed. If you are satisfied with whatever the hospital has done or offered, then settle the matter. If you are not or you are not sure especially if you or your loved one has been seriously injured, you may want to consult an attorney.

## When to Sue Over OOPs!

After having reviewed many cases of potential medical malpractice over the years as a medical expert, a hospitalist group leader, or National Medical Director for the country's largest hospitalist group, I've seen that these cases usually fall into one of three groups: Obvious errors or missed diagnoses, unfortunate outcomes that caused harm but were not necessarily due to errors, and cases that are between these two.

Interestingly, having evaluated many cases, I also see that most patients are motivated to sue by more than the promise of compensation. For example, while my mother chose not to sue after her botched foot surgery, she wanted the doctor to acknowledge and apologize for his mistake.

Many patients just want respect. To show this respect, some hospitals are experimenting with complete transparency. For example, the University of Michigan has a policy to divulge and apologize for all medical errors as soon as they are discovered, even if the patient might never know about the error. Sometimes the hospital even includes patients and their families in root-cause analysis meant to discover the sources of these errors. Of course, admitting errors leads to the hospital having to pay for extra care and procedures to fix these things, but it can also lead to fewer settlements and court cases down the line.

Know that if you choose to sue, it can be difficult to win. A 2009 study that examined 20 years of legal rulings found that doctors win 80–90 percent of jury cases with weak evidence, 70 percent of borderline cases and patients still win only 50 percent of cases even with strong evidence of medical negligence. With OOPs, prevention is best. Working with your insurance company and maybe your hospital or doctor is next. Then if needed you can explore patient advocacy. I am not about to give legal advice but follow your gut and ask yourself what you really want. If it feels like the right thing to do and legal experts agree that you have a very strong case, you may want to pursue legal action. I have advised all of the above depending on the situation.

# CHAPTER 23:
## Negotiating Your Own Deals

O nce upon a time there were four quarterbacks, each in a different quadrant of value. One was named Peyton Manning and another was named Ryan Leaf. They were the #1 and #2 picks in the 1998 NFL draft, going to the Colts and Chargers respectively. Both of these highly touted quarterbacks were very expensive, making in the realm of $20 million each for their first years in the league. Manning went on to win a Super Bowl with the Colts and another with Denver and could be the greatest quarterback of all time. Ryan Leaf is considered one of the greatest draft-pick flops of all time, not only failing as a quarterback but also ending up in jail. Manning was in the high-cost/high-quality quadrant of value. Leaf was in the high-cost/low-quality quadrant.

Two years later, two more quarterbacks entered the league. Tom Brady went to the Patriots with the 199th pick and Todd Husak went to the Redskins with pick number 202. Their first year, Brady made about $250,000 and Husak made about $400,000. In the NFL, both were cheap. You probably know how Tom Brady turned out. And Husak played three NFL plays for a net -3 yards. Brady was in the low-cost/high-quality quadrant and Husak was in the low-cost/low-quality quadrant (Husak has since gone on to earn an advanced degree from Stanford and is a very successful businessman, but I had to pick someone in the low/low quadrant...sorry, Todd).

This makes Brady the poster child for what every team wants: low cost and high quality make very high value. All healthcare teams want to make Tom-Brady–like choices. Unless you have an infinitely heavy pocketbook, you want to make these high-value choices too. But the fact of the matter is, your healthcare may not start out in this high-value quadrant. In order to get the most from your healthcare dollar, you may need to negotiate. This chapter is your primer to being your own agent when negotiating your healthcare bills. The most important thing to know is that you *can*. When it comes to medical bills, you have options. Actually, you have exactly five options: Use your insurance and don't negotiate; use your insurance but negotiate the portion you owe; pay cash without negotiating; negotiate the bill and pay cash for the remaining amount; bid for healthcare before you use it. Let's look at these options now.

## Use Your Insurance Without Negotiating

Let's say your insurer has signed a contract to pay your doctor $3,500 to perform a colonoscopy. After study, you offer your doctor $1,000 cash for the procedure. Because cash is king in healthcare, there's a pretty good chance your doctor will accept. The only problem is, you've outsmarted yourself.

With insurance, your portion of the colonoscopy is exactly $0. Despite what sounds like a big price tag, you can't be charged a cent. When choosing whether to negotiate healthcare costs, first make sure you're not negotiating against yourself. Understand *your part of the bill*. There's a chance it will look much better than the overall price tag—that's why you pay your monthly premium! And there's a good chance the overall price tag already represents the result of negotiations between your provider and your insurance company. Make sure you understand your real costs before you jump into negotiations.

## Negotiate Your Portion of the Bill

If you have private insurance (not Medicare or Medicaid) and you know that you will need a surgery or procedure, you can call ahead to negotiate a discount on your part of the bill. This is especially useful if you are still paying toward your deductible. As you might expect, it is always best to do this negotiating before the service. But even if you open your mailbox to find an OOPs bill from your insurance staring you in the face, it's worth calling to see what can be done about your portion. That is, unless your insurance is Medicare or Medicaid. People on these government plans are not allowed to negotiate the cost of their care.

## Paying Cash

Let's check off the most unlikely scenario: if you're paying cash, why would you not see if you can negotiate a lower price? Maybe a better question than whether you should negotiate when paying cash is when you should pay cash in the first place. First, if you are in one of the new models like an ACO, Patient

Centered Medical Home, or a bundled procedure you may not be allowed to pay cash—you may be required to use your insurance. Ask your insurance company about these restrictions.

Then, probably the most common scenario of paying cash for healthcare is if you have a high deductible insurance plan. If you are on the hook for $1,000 or $5,000 or more before your insurance even kicks in, it's worth taking a close look at the price of the CAT scan ordered by the ER after you got beaned during the office softball party. On the low end, it could cost only $300 and on the high end, you could end up meeting your high deductible this year, after all. That said, if you are billed for care by your high-deductible plan, your insurance company has *already* negotiated the price. The cost on your bill represents your insurance company's agreement with your hospital or doctor. It's still worth checking, but you may not be able to negotiate a further reduction.

It's when you *don't* have insurance that the real cash negotiations begin. And let's reiterate a point from this book's first section: Since 2014, the ACA has mandated that you have health insurance. Okay, let's say you still don't have insurance. Now let's say you need a CAT scan. It's not out of the question to end up with a $4,000 bill. If you're able to negotiate this price ahead of time, great. If you have to negotiate the cost after, that's okay but still do-able in most situations. Just remember that it's probably not best to negotiate *during* a procedure.

## How to Negotiate a Cash Price

In order to negotiate, you need to know how much things are likely to cost. Check websites like Healthcarebluebook.com and Clearhealthcarecosts.com to see how much wiggle room you should expect in a hospital's stated price. These sites are very general and do not take into account variations in quality between hospitals/providers but can be a great way to get a big picture idea of the cost side of value.

Once you have a general idea how much a procedure should cost, compare it to your salary cap. How much can you realistically afford? Knowing this number could help you negotiate toward a manageable fee or it could help you make the decision to get creative. When getting creative, remember that you have more than one choice of facility and doctor. If one doctor won't go below your salary cap, consider working with another. Remember that procedures in a surgery center or doctor's office may be less expensive than the same procedure in a hospital.

When calling a doctor's office, ask to speak with the practice manager or business manager. If you're calling a surgery center, let the receptionist know you're considering a procedure and then ask to speak with the business manager or chief financial officer. At a hospital, start at the top by letting them know you're considering a procedure and would like to speak with the chief financial officer. Expect to be referred to someone lower on the food chain.

Then when you reach the right person, ask what is their preferred method of payment for a discount? Chances are it's cash, but some hospitals have worked out special deals with certain credit cards. If at all possible, offer to pay upfront and in full—this will give you far and away the most leverage. Also, make sure that the hospital knows you will not be using insurance and that you will be paying 100 percent out of your pocket. When you get an offer, get it in writing. Make sure you also list the person who offered you this price—get the name, position, and contact information.

Finally, consider bundling the costs of your procedure. Ask for a bundle to include everything—anesthesia, facility fees, and even follow-up visits. If you are negotiating the price of a surgery or procedure, you can also ask that any complications be fixed without additional cost.

Do not pay the bill until you get the entire itemized invoice, not just the statement. This allows the opposite of bundling— you may be able to reduce or remove the cost of certain line items, especially if you or your family kept an accurate log of your treatments. You can also double-check that you are not charged for routine services, like a ventilator in the ICU, which should be part of the facility's daily charge, or a nurse who checks your blood glucose, which should be part of the nursing charge.

Now that you've brought the bill down as much as possible through "normal" channels, if the cost remains above your salary cap, it's worth talking to someone face-to-face (especially if you're the type of person who can speak calmly without losing your temper). Ask about charity assistance or sliding scale payments. If at all possible, offer a lump-sum payment on the spot. Hospitals may cut the bill substantially if they are paid right away. If this is not possible you can set up a payment plan, which in many cases will prevent a provider from turning you over to a collection agency.

In the end, negotiating is about leverage. What leverage do you have as a "little old me"? You don't have the leverage provided by representing a huge number of people with a giant number of dollars. But you do have the leverage of promising to be quick and easy (or their opposite). Doctors value time and lack of hassle. To a degree, they may even value ease of payment over amount of payment. This is your leverage.

## Bidding and Bartering: Out-of-the-Box Healthcare Payment Solutions

I once treated an HIV+ patient who had no health insurance. Over the years, he had many complications and hospitalizations, and his partner wanted to use his artistic skills to pay me back for the care I gave. Once we were talking and when he learned we were repainting our living room, he asked if he could paint the ceiling for us. I reluctantly agreed and he painted with the love and skill of Michelangelo decorating the Sistine Chapel, at least that's what it looked like to me. When he was done, I insisted on paying him…so I guess it wasn't a trade after all. But every time I walked into that room I thought of my patient and the appreciation he and his partner had for my care. The honor was mine.

Believe it or not you can trade or barter for healthcare. You can barter directly with your doctor or, more commonly, you can go through an exchange, earning some kind of unit credit or virtual currency for your services. You can then turn around and "spend" this virtual currency on healthcare. On the Florida Bartering website, you can barter for everything from disc jockeys for your next party to doctors for your next colonoscopy!

Or, websites like Medibid allow you to bid for procedures. If a doctor accepts your price, you are matched and may move forward. Of course, because any registered provider can accept your bid, you have only the cost and not the quality information needed to make a value judgment. As the philosophies that control the government change, expect new avenues to make deals and contracts with doctors. Even Medicare patients may earn the ability to negotiate, contracting directly with doctors regardless of whether they participate in the plan.

And in my opinion, here is the big danger with these out-of-the-box payment solutions: With bidding and bartering, will you end up only with healthcare options from the low-low quadrant of value—low cost and low quality? After setting up your barter or having your bid accepted, do your homework to ensure the care you're buying is care you want.

# CHAPTER 24:
## Medicines are your Offensive Weapons

For a number of years after high school my older sister, Laura, and I had a symbiotic arrangement: she dated my friends and I dated hers. Before my freshman year of college, we planned one last tubing trip down the Guadalupe River in Kerr County, Texas—I brought my friend, Chip, and Laura brought her friend, Dawn. With the drinking age at 18, we loaded a cooler with tallboys and secured it in the most seaworthy tube, figuring that we could swim but the beers could not. Priorities straight, we hit the river: the air was hot, the water was cold, and the beer was even colder. What could go wrong?

Tethered together, we floated down the river, stopping at a rope swing where I executed a flawless back-flop to the joy and jeers of everyone on the river. My sister's tube came loose from our flotilla and bumped the shore before she was able to fight her way back into the current. When she closed her eyes and leaned back, we thought she was soaking in the sun. The more we laughed, the more she withdrew. Finally she moaned, "I don't feel right…" before her eyes lolled back in her head and she passed out, her head falling in the water over the side of her tube.

Chip and I raced to her and pulled her head from the water, but she didn't respond. We shook her and screamed, but she didn't wake up. Becoming a doctor was still years away and I had no idea what to do. Thank God there were campers who heard the commotion and as we struggled to shore, they pulled up with a pickup truck. "There's a hospital not far from here!" the driver yelled as Chip and I tossed my sister in the open back and jumped in after her. We started mouth-to-mouth, but didn't know how many breaths or when to check a pulse. Laura's face was red and swollen, a rash creeping over her chest. We were only two beers into the afternoon—was it a seizure or a stroke? I was pretty sure she was going to die. The driver took the rutted roads at Mach 3.

"Where is that hospital?" I yelled. I started to think about what I would tell our mother. Finally we screamed up to the ER and a nurse came running out with a stretcher, meeting us halfway to the door as a doctor began to bark orders. I struggled to fill him in: "We were on the river…she started to have trouble breathing…she was turning blue and rolled over…we raced here! No, she only had two beers and we were only 45 minutes into the trip. Is she going to make it?"

He yelled for epinephrine and I started to make deals with God. After what seemed like an eternity he came out to tell us she was responding to treatment. She was going to make it. Later we learned that she had a deadly allergy to fire ants, the scourge of Texas summers. She'd been bitten when her tube touched the shore, but didn't think anything of it. When we left for college that next week, she to Penn State and me to

University of Texas at Austin, we hugged just a little bit longer and just a little bit tighter.

Drugs save lives. Sometimes it's in the emergency setting like that day on the river with my sister, sometimes it's a medication to cure a condition like cancer or antibiotics to fight and infection or a daily medication to improve health or keep a chronic condition at bay. But the fact remains: drugs save lives.

Like a great quarterback, medications can be a healthcare team's best offensive weapon. But we don't have the NFL's billions and so too often we also have to take into account the cost of these medications. The skyrocketing price and cost of pharmaceuticals is no longer sustainable. I can't tell you how many times I've had the following conversation.

*Me:* "Did you keep taking your medication after you left the hospital?"

*Patient:* "To tell the truth, no, Doc. When the pharmacist told me how much it was I never filled the prescription."

According to a Kaiser Family Foundation survey, 24 percent of patients report not filling a prescription and 19 percent say they cut pills in half or skipped a dose due to cost. Overall, up to 33 percent had trouble affording medications. A *Consumer Reports* survey showed it's not getting better with one-third of people reporting a spike in prescription drugs costs in the past year.

So the question is not only which offensive weapon you should use for your condition, but how to pay for it? How can you find value in medications? Here are some rules to follow:

## Ditching Unneeded Medications Is the Best Value of All

Everything has a possible side effect: eating peanuts can be deadly, jewelry can cause a blistering rash, and even too much oxygen can be bad. Just as even the smallest surgery carries risk, so does every medication—and the decision process for choosing to start a medication should be the same as that for surgery. Do you need it? Do you want it? Can you afford it? What are the benefits and what are the risks?

Antibiotics are at the forefront of the want/need debate. Let's take a common scenario: you bring your child to his or her pediatrician with a bad cold. But colds and ear infections and sinus infections and bronchitis can all be viral as opposed to bacterial infections. Of course, antibiotics only kill bacteria and not viruses. There are some tests your doctor can perform to determine if viruses or bacteria are to blame...but then, even if the doctor thinks your child has a viral infection, so many parents ask for antibiotics and so many doctors prescribe them.

This is a losing strategy. Why? First, antibiotics can harm your child. Forget about allergies and diarrhea caused by antibiotics—killing off your good gut bacteria can allow bad gut bacteria to grow. I once took care of a 45-year-old woman who needed to be admitted to the ICU after taking a few antibiotics before and after her gallbladder surgery. The surgery had gone well and she was otherwise healthy, but her antibiotics had allowed the bacteria C. *difficile* to populate her gut. She survived, but it wasn't good.

In an obvious TEAM vs. "me" conflict, taking an unneeded antibiotic may be only a little bit bad for you, but a population of people taking unneeded antibiotics is terrible for society. Over time, as a bacteria is exposed to an antibiotic it can learn how to outsmart it. American doctors giving too many antibiotics have created a breeding ground for super-bugs. The result is the recent finding of a strain of E. *coli* (a common bacteria) that is resistant to our most powerful antibiotics. If you think your bacterial pneumonia is hard to treat now, just wait 20 years. Some other drugs work this way too—using something now may make it work less well later.

One reason for the overprescription of antibiotics is a disconnect in the shared decision-making between doctor and patient. I have had patients tell me they will never get better without an antibiotic. "Trust me," they say, "I have had this for years and every time I need an antibiotic." I try to suggest that the patient might have gotten better without an antibiotic, that it may be time to break the cycle, that I think they have a viral infection. But the opinion of antibiotics as a super drug is hard to break. Doctors sometimes don't have the time or will to talk patients out of their desire for antibiotics. It doesn't help that doctors may be scored on patient experience surveys and may not want to generate an angry result.

Don't put yourself and society at risk by insisting on unneeded antibiotics or any other medicine that sounds good but turns out to have no benefit.

## Polypharmacy in the Elderly

An NFL team can never have too many offensive weapons but that is not true for medications. According to Medscape, patients aged 65–84 fill an average of 14–18 prescriptions per year. Not only is this expensive, but each new medicine creates the chance for a bad reaction or interaction. This had led to a movement to de-prescribe. When you and your doctor determine that a new medication has value, use it as an opportunity to review your current medications to see if any on the list are value-less. Take this chance to de-prescribe.

As Gordon Schiff wrote in the *New England Journal of Medicine*, one useful tool toward de-prescription of medicines that are no longer needed would be for doctors to include *reasons* with their prescriptions. How many times have you picked up a prescription at the pharmacy with a name you don't remember in the least? What was that for again? Oh well, your doctor probably said you should have it and so you fill the prescription with no other questions. Having a drug's indication along with a drug's name and dosing would allow you to evaluate its usefulness. Is it really worth paying $179 for a heartburn pill or could you ditch the drug and decide that your jalapeno days are behind you?

## Remember Transitions

When you are transitioning across facilities and teams make sure to double-check your medications list. Doctors call this "medication reconciliation." I've always found this term a little funny—did the medications not get along? Of course, medication reconciliation is the process that brings what you *have* been taking into line with what you *will* be taking. This is another excellent time to confirm your need for each medication on your list.

## Generics Drugs Are the Tom Bradys of Healthcare

Remember the four quadrants of value? There's low-cost/low-quality, high-cost/high-quality, high-cost/low-quality… and then there's Tom Brady, the low-cost/high-quality diamond in the rough. Actually, Brady *used* to be the low-high epitome of value, making $250,000 during his first years in the league.

You better bet he makes a bit more than that now, landing him in the high-high value quadrant. Drugs in America do the opposite. They start out in the high-cost/high-quality value quadrant but when they go off patent, they can move into that low-cost/high-value, "Tom Brady" quadrant. That is, if there is a company willing to invest in manufacturing a generic drug that can pass all the hurdles of the Food and Drug Administration (FDA). If you could get Tom Brady on the cheap, why wouldn't you? Usually doctors will offer a generic alternative when one exists—if your doctor forgets or if you're staring at a prescription for a drug that pushes the upper end of your salary cap, consider asking if there's a generic alternative. In fact, a study in JAMA found that American healthcare could have saved $73 billion dollars had it used generic drugs whenever possible from 2010–2012. For you, that's a lot of OOPs!

The lower cost of generics is true even if you're using insurance. According to the 2015 Kaiser Family Foundation Employer Survey for Market Place Plans the average insurance co-pay for generic drugs was $12.23, for preferred brands (like an in-network drug) it was $44.72, for non-preferred brands it was $87.07, and for specialty drugs the co-pay was $252.38. Some insurances even penalize you for buying name-brand drugs when a generic is available!

## Check with Your Insurance First

If you need an inexpensive medicine, you can fill the prescription knowing that even if your insurance happens for some reason to refuse payment, you're only out a couple bucks. But some drugs are just plain expensive. Take Soliris, used to treat a couple dangerous blood diseases—its annual cost is about $440,000. That's a bill you'll want to make sure your insurance is covering. Do it before the bill shows up in the mail. With a new expensive medication, play prevent defense—check with your insurance to make sure it will be covered.

## The Middle Men

One of the most rewarding weeks of my life was a medical mission to Haiti, organized by my church. Three doctors, several nurses, and a handful of volunteers were met at the Port au Prince airport by a priest named Father Bruni, who had organized our clinic. Unfortunately, after going through customs we realized that airport officials had seized all of our medications and supplies. I don't know what he said or what he did, but Father Bruni talked to several different officials and the next thing we knew, the meds and supplies were being loaded into our Jeep.

Most insurers and employers use the medical equivalent to Father Bruni, companies called Pharmacy Benefit Managers (PBMs), which act as middlemen between patients/employees and medications. When you use your insurance, you will have to play by the rules of these middlemen. They determine the drugs that your doctor can prescribe and what "tier" or price you will have to pay. When an inexpensive drug offers obvious benefit, TEAM and "me" align and the PBM is your best friend, negotiating the best prices from drug companies and pharmacies on the behalf of your insurance company (who, one hopes, passes on these savings to you). When a more expensive drug offers less clear benefit, TEAM and "me" can misalign and the PBM is more like the officials who held the medications. When a drug is below a PBM's value threshold, it's this middleman that can refuse to cover it.

## Shopping for the Best Medication Price

All it takes is a couple clicks to find a fly-by-night website selling discount meds manufactured overseas. But ask yourself: Are you willing to gamble with your health? When shopping around for meds, make sure online sites display the seal of a Verified Internet Pharmacy Practice Site (VIPPS). A good place to start is GoodRx.com. Also check drug prices on the websites of pharmacies like Walgreens, CVS, and Costco. Now armed with the best published prices, don't forget to negotiate! Using your best agent voice, ask, "Is this your best price, because I found it lower across the street!" Stores will often match a lower price.

## If You Cannot Afford Your Medications

You are not alone. Many Americans struggling to pay rent and put food on the table face a tough choice: do you want to eat or buy meds? This terrible dilemma is one reason I am a co-leader of the Doctors for America Drug Price Value and Affordability Campaign. In fact, our petition in collaboration with other groups led to the drug company Mylan offering a generic for EpiPen. I will continue to fight this battle. Until drug prices come down or your salary goes up, consider asking your doctor for samples of your medication. Remember, these samples won't last forever, but these meds lying around your doctor's office can tide you over until you can make a better plan. Also, ask how you can get in touch with the company that makes the medication you need. Sometimes you can work with their patient assistance program to bring down the price. Programs exist for needy patients—don't just assume that because a medication's published price is way over your salary cap that the drug is unattainable.

Unfortunately, not all stories of expensive medications have a happy ending. Despite her allergies and the potential risk, my sister has decided that the price of EpiPen is too high to justify the purchase and has stopped carrying one. This calculation is a very personal choice—what is your health worth?

The following are all great resources for prescription assistance:

## FreeDrugCard.us

Nationwide Prescription Assistance Program (PAP) sponsored by a *non-profit organization* to help all Americans lower their prescription drug costs. This program has *LOWEST PRICE LOGIC* to guarantee that you get the best deal on your prescriptions.

## PPARx.org

The Partnership for Prescription Assistance brings together America's pharmaceutical companies, doctors, other health-care providers, patient advocacy organizations, and community groups to help qualifying patients who lack prescription coverage get the medicines they need through the public or private program that's right for them.

## TogetherRxAccess.com

The Together Rx Access Program can help millions of Americans, who have no prescription drug coverage and are not eligible for Medicare, save on prescription products. Most cardholders save 25% to 40% on brand-name prescription drugs and products.

## Needymeds.com

This Web site gives information about PAPs. The site also lists drugs that are available through PAPs and gives contact information for the companies that make them.

## RxHope.com

This site is supported by the Pharmaceutical Research and Manufacturers of America (also called PhRMA). Using the tools on the RxHope site, your doctor can apply for you to receive free or low-cost drugs from the companies that make them.

## Rxassist.org

This Web site is sponsored by an organization called Volunteers in Health Care. By searching the database on this website, you or your doctor, nurse, or social worker can find out which PAPs you might qualify for.

I hope that my *Healthcare Playbook* helps you to navigate your own healthcare journey for yourselves and your loved ones. This journey, like football, can be filled with fumbles, interceptions, and missed play calls. Winning the modern game of medicine is different for everyone but it starts with you being the MVP, the center of care. Be empowered and informed, know when you have choice and maximize it to get the most value. Watch the **"teams of teams"** in healthcare and make sure they put **"ME"** or **"You"** above the teams. I wish you only touchdowns for your health, the most important game of your life!